Surgical Manual of Implant Dentistry:
Step-By-Step Procedures

Surgical Manual of Implant Dentistry
Step-By-Step Procedures

Daniel Buser, DDS, Dr med dent
Professor and Chairman
Department of Oral Surgery and Stomatology
School of Dental Medicine
University of Bern
Bern, Switzerland

Jun-Young Cho, DDS
Associate Professor
Department of Periodontics
Baylor College of Dentistry
Texas A & M University System Health Science Center
Dallas, Texas

Alvin B. K. Yeo, BDS, MSc
Periodontics Unit
Department of Restorative Dentistry
National Dental Centre
Republic of Singapore

Quintessence Publishing Co, Inc

Chicago, Berlin, Tokyo, London, Paris, Milan, Barcelona, Istanbul, São Paulo,
Mumbai, Moscow, Prague, and Warsaw

Library of Congress Cataloging-in-Publication Data

Buser, Daniel.
  Surgical manual of implant dentistry : step-by-step procedures /
Daniel Buser, Jun Y. Cho, Alvin Yeo.
    p. ; cm.
  ISBN-13: 978-0-86715-379-8
  1. Dental implants--Handbooks, manuals, etc. 2. Dental implants
--Atlases.   I. Cho, Jun Y. II. Yeo, Alvin. III. Title.
  [DNLM: 1. Dental Implantation--methods--Atlases. 2. Dental
Implantation--methods--Case Reports.   WU 600.7 B977s 2007]
RK667.I45S874 2007
617.6'93--dc22

                                   2006033380

© 2007 Quintessence Publishing Co, Inc

Quintessence Publishing Co, Inc
4350 Chandler Drive
Hanover Park, Illinois 60133
www.quintpub.com

Editor: Bryn Goates
Design and production: Dawn Hartman

Printed in Canada

Table of Contents

Preface

Based on the concept of osseointegration first described by Brånemark and Schroeder, implant dentistry has evolved tremendously over the past 15 years, and today it plays an integral role in dental rehabilitation. Though it was developed primarily to rehabilitate fully edentulous patients, since the late 1980s the treatment focus has gradually shifted to partially edentulous patients. Today, single-tooth replacement is the number one indication for implant therapy.

Implant dentistry also has benefited from the significant progress made in associated treatment protocols. Development of bone augmentation procedures allows clinicians to correct alveolar bone deficiencies, while guided bone regeneration with barrier membranes and sinus floor elevation have become standards of care to correct bone defects in other parts of the oral cavity. In addition, improved osteophilic microtextured titanium implant surfaces help to accelerate healing, significantly reducing treatment time. Together, these advances make implant therapy more predictable and more attractive to patients, and the result has been a rapid expansion of implant dentistry in daily practice and more clinicians placing dental implants.

This book is the culmination of many years' effort to standardize surgical technique in implant dentistry. It is designed for postdoctoral students and practitioners who wish to perform surgical implant procedures in daily practice with a high predictability for success and a low risk for complications. Basic surgical principles and procedures for placing implants both in standard sites and in sites with local defects are presented using detailed explanations and hand-drawn illustrations. The final chapter of the book presents 14 comprehensive clinical case reports, several documenting long-term follow-ups over a period of 10 years.

The publication of this book coincides with the production of a DVD featuring live surgery of the same surgical techniques in seven clinical cases. The surgery was recorded during master courses in implant dentistry offered by the University of Bern.

The authors wish to thank the staff of Quintessence Publishing for their excellent support during the preparation and production of this book.

Basic Surgical Principles

This chapter presents the basic surgical principles related to the placement of Straumann implants in partially edentulous patients. To achieve successful osseointegration, a precise and low-trauma surgical technique is required. Surgeons must take important measures preoperatively to prevent postsurgical infection, handle surgical instruments expertly to preserve soft tissues, and carefully accomplish adequate implant site preparation without overheating the bone. Precise surgical protocol includes the following precautions:

- Preoperative mouthwash with 0.1% chlorhexidine
- Perioral skin disinfection with alcohol solution
- Antibiotic prophylaxis 2 hours prior to surgery (eg, 2 g amoxicillin intraorally)
- Low-speed drilling (between 500 and 600 rpm)
- Cooling spray during drilling with chilled sterile saline
- Intermittent drilling technique
- Use of sharp drills

It is important to perform a surgical procedure systematically, always applying the same surgical principles.

Fig 1-1   Smoothing the alveolar crest following flap elevation.

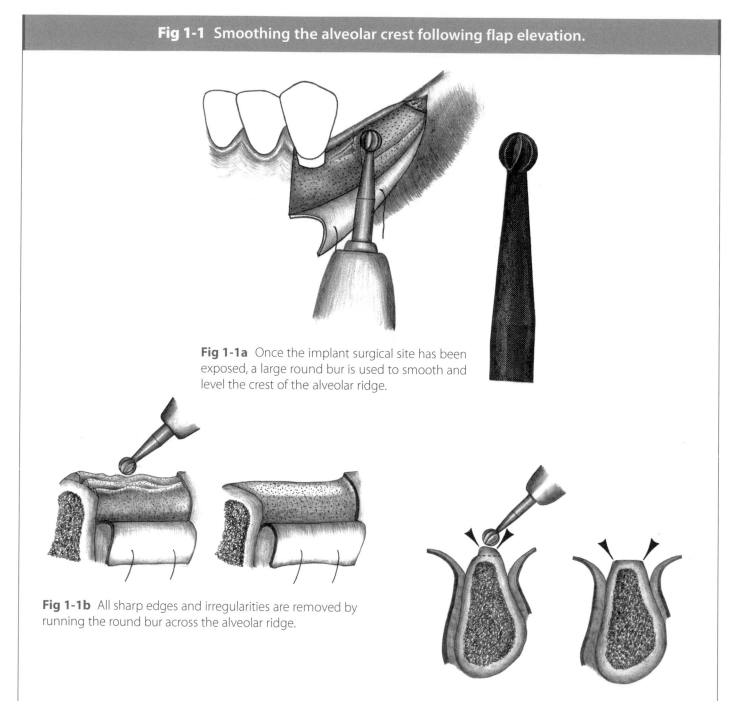

Fig 1-1a Once the implant surgical site has been exposed, a large round bur is used to smooth and level the crest of the alveolar ridge.

Fig 1-1b All sharp edges and irregularities are removed by running the round bur across the alveolar ridge.

Fig 1-1c In this cross section, the irregular, narrow crest is smoothed to produce a flat, wide ridge, which is favorable for implant site preparation.

Fig 1-2 Sequence of site preparation for a standard implant.

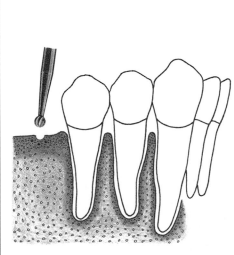

Fig 1-2a A no. 1 round bur is used to mark the position of the implant site.

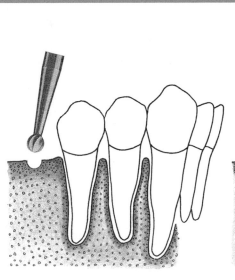

Fig 1-2b Access is widened with a no. 2 round bur. This step makes it possible to correctly position the next drill.

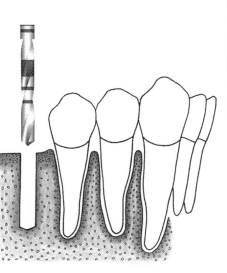

Fig 1-2c The initial implant site preparation is made with a 2.2-mm-diameter pilot drill.

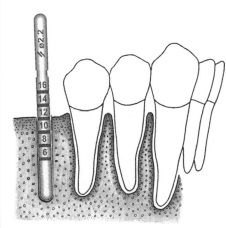

Fig 1-2d A 2.2-mm-diameter guide pin is inserted into the initial preparation to check its position and axis.

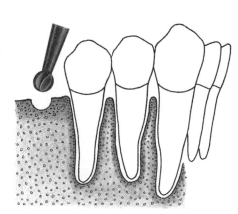

Fig 1-2e The crest of the osteotomy is enlarged with a no. 3 round bur.

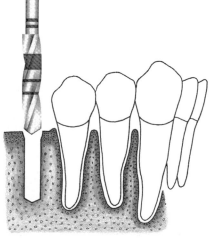

Fig 1-2f A 2.8-mm-diameter spiral drill is easily inserted for preparing the depth of the site.

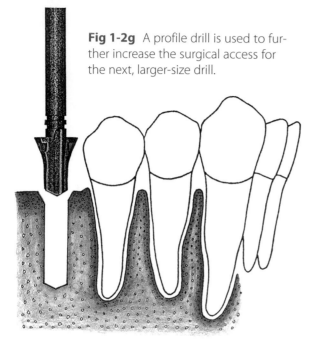

Fig 1-2g A profile drill is used to further increase the surgical access for the next, larger-size drill.

Fig 1-2h Preparation of the implant site continues with the 3.5-mm-diameter spiral drill.

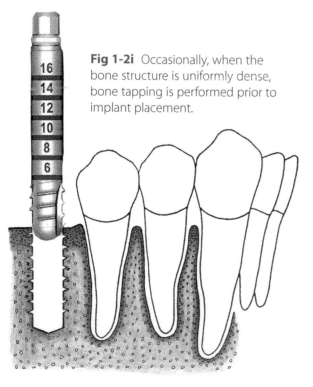

Fig 1-2i Occasionally, when the bone structure is uniformly dense, bone tapping is performed prior to implant placement.

Fig 1-2j A standard implant is placed in the site, with the rough surface positioned at the level of the alveolar ridge crest. This allows the implant shoulder to be located at the gingival level.

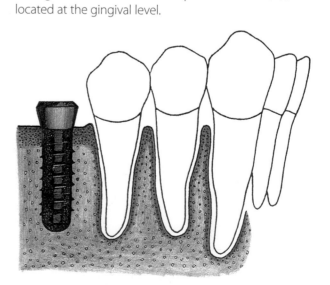

Fig 1-3 Correction of the position and axis of the implant site preparation.

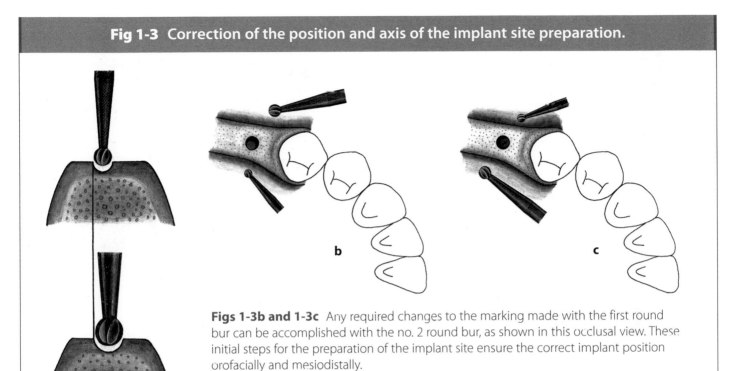

Figs 1-3b and 1-3c Any required changes to the marking made with the first round bur can be accomplished with the no. 2 round bur, as shown in this occlusal view. These initial steps for the preparation of the implant site ensure the correct implant position orofacially and mesiodistally.

Fig 1-3a The preparation of the implant site begins with the use of the nos. 1 and 2 round burs to mark the position of the implant site.

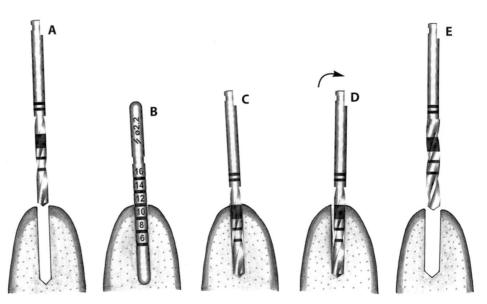

Fig 1-3d After the use of the first pilot drill *(A)*, a 2.2-mm-diameter guide pin is used to check the axis and depth of the implant preparation *(B)*. Any incorrect axis orientation can be adjusted with the same 2.2-mm-diameter pilot drill *(C and D)* and then followed with the 2.8-mm-diameter spiral drill *(E)*.

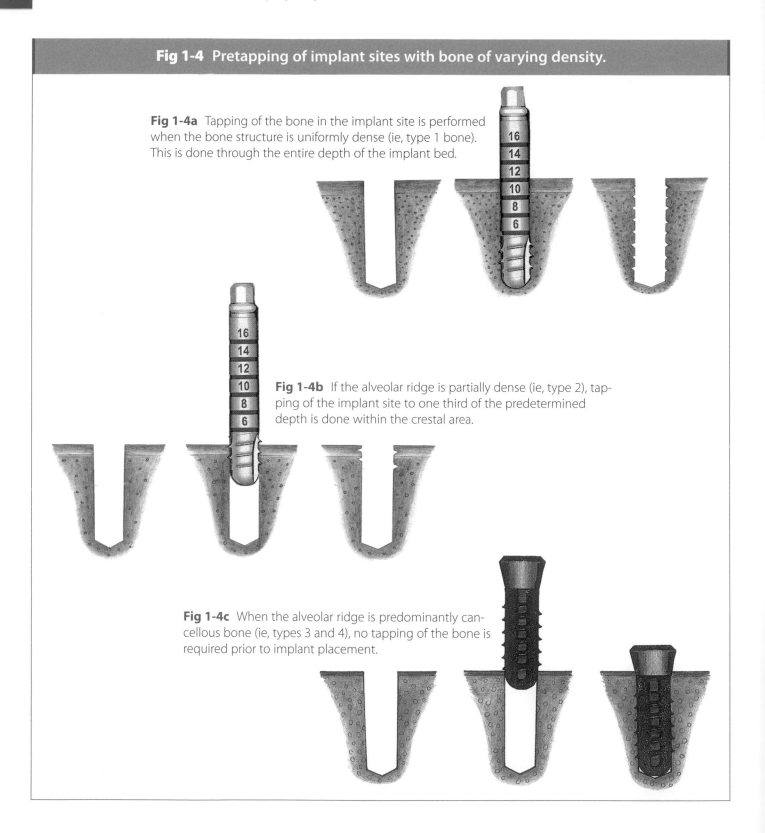

Fig 1-4 **Pretapping of implant sites with bone of varying density.**

Fig 1-4a Tapping of the bone in the implant site is performed when the bone structure is uniformly dense (ie, type 1 bone). This is done through the entire depth of the implant bed.

Fig 1-4b If the alveolar ridge is partially dense (ie, type 2), tapping of the implant site to one third of the predetermined depth is done within the crestal area.

Fig 1-4c When the alveolar ridge is predominantly cancellous bone (ie, types 3 and 4), no tapping of the bone is required prior to implant placement.

Fig 1-5 Varying sink depths.

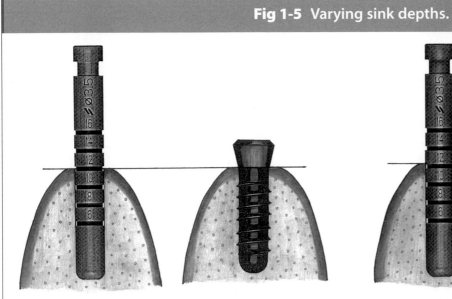

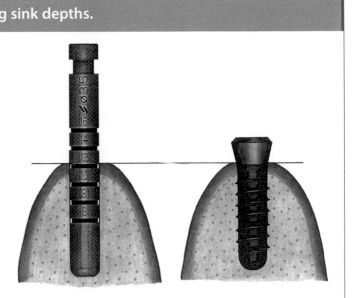

Fig 1-5a The 3.5-mm-diameter depth gauge is inserted so that the middle of the 12-mm mark is aligned with the bone crest *(left)*. When the standard implant is inserted, this allows the rough border to be aligned exactly at the crest *(right)*.

Fig 1-5b If the implant site is prepared with the 12-mm mark slightly below the crest, the rough border of the inserted implant will be positioned approximately 0.5 mm below the crest. This approach is most often used in posterior implant sites for a nonsubmerged implant healing.

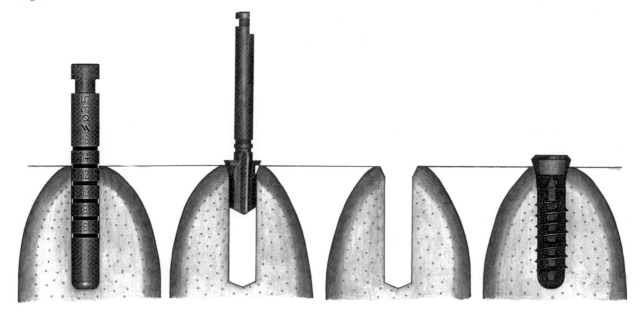

Fig 1-5c The implant site is prepared to the 14-mm mark, and the profile drill is used to flare the coronal portion of the crest. A 12-mm-long standard implant can be inserted more deeply to partially submerge the machined collar. This approach is normally used in esthetic implant sites for a submerged implant healing.

Fig 1-6 Overview of implant site preparation and implant placement.

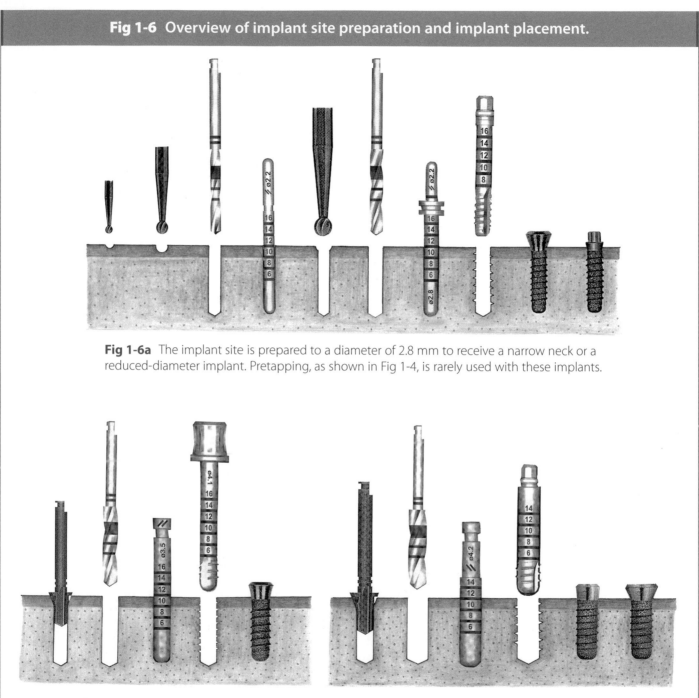

Fig 1-6a The implant site is prepared to a diameter of 2.8 mm to receive a narrow neck or a reduced-diameter implant. Pretapping, as shown in Fig 1-4, is rarely used with these implants.

Fig 1-6b When a standard implant is used, the implant site is prepared to a diameter of 3.5 mm. Pretapping, as shown in Fig 1-4, is rarely used.

Fig 1-6c The implant site is prepared to a diameter of 4.2 mm, and a wide body or wide neck implant is inserted. Pretapping, as shown in Fig 1-4, is used more often due to larger implant diameter.

Fig 1-7 Selection of implant length in the posterior mandible.

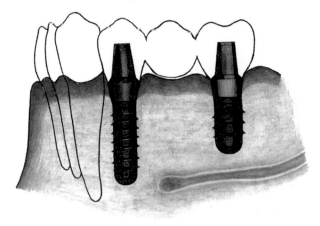

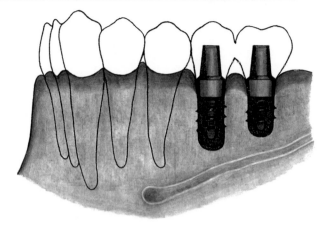

Fig 1-7a In regions restricted by anatomic limitations, shorter implants are frequently used. In this long-span mandibular distal extension situation, two implants are placed to support a three-unit fixed partial denture. An 8-mm short implant *(right)* is used to avoid the mandibular canal.

Fig 1-7b In a short-span mandibular distal extension situation, two short implants with lengths of 6 and/or 8 mm may be indicated. They are used here to avoid the mandibular canal. These short implants are often restored with splinted crowns.

Fig 1-8 Selection of implant length in the posterior maxilla.

Fig 1-8 In the maxillary posterior distal extension situation, the maxillary sinus can be avoided with the use of shorter implants. Here, two implants (12 and 8 mm) are inserted in the second premolar and first molar sites, respectively, in close proximity to the sinus.

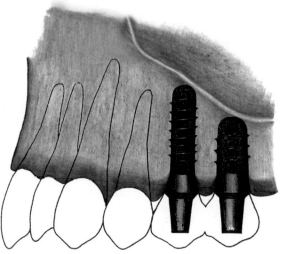

Fig 1-9 Minimum width of alveolar crest for implants of varying diameter.

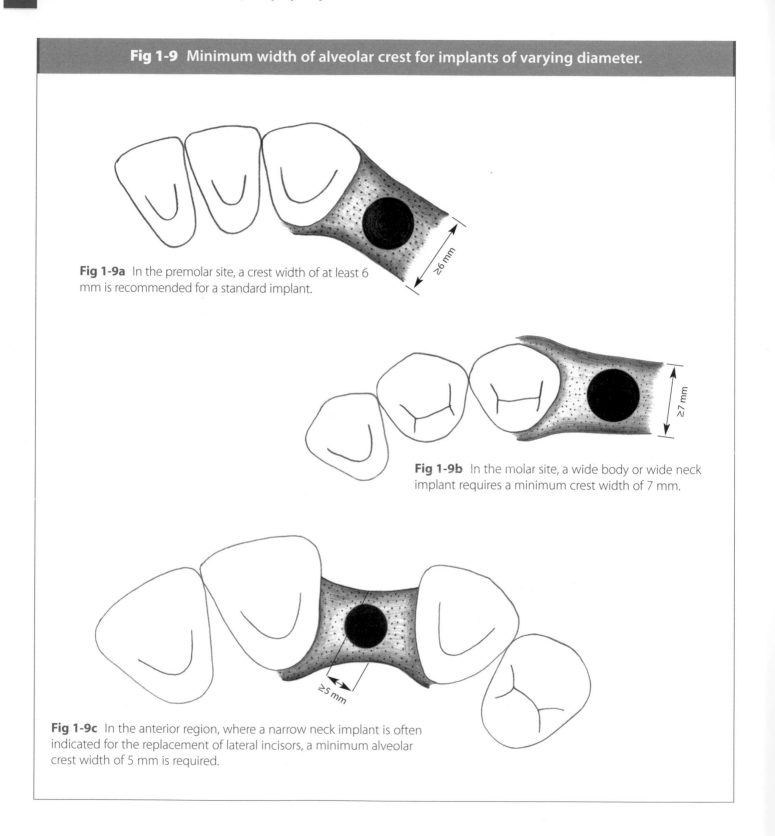

Fig 1-9a In the premolar site, a crest width of at least 6 mm is recommended for a standard implant.

Fig 1-9b In the molar site, a wide body or wide neck implant requires a minimum crest width of 7 mm.

Fig 1-9c In the anterior region, where a narrow neck implant is often indicated for the replacement of lateral incisors, a minimum alveolar crest width of 5 mm is required.

Fig 1-10 Minimum space of single-tooth gaps for various implant types.

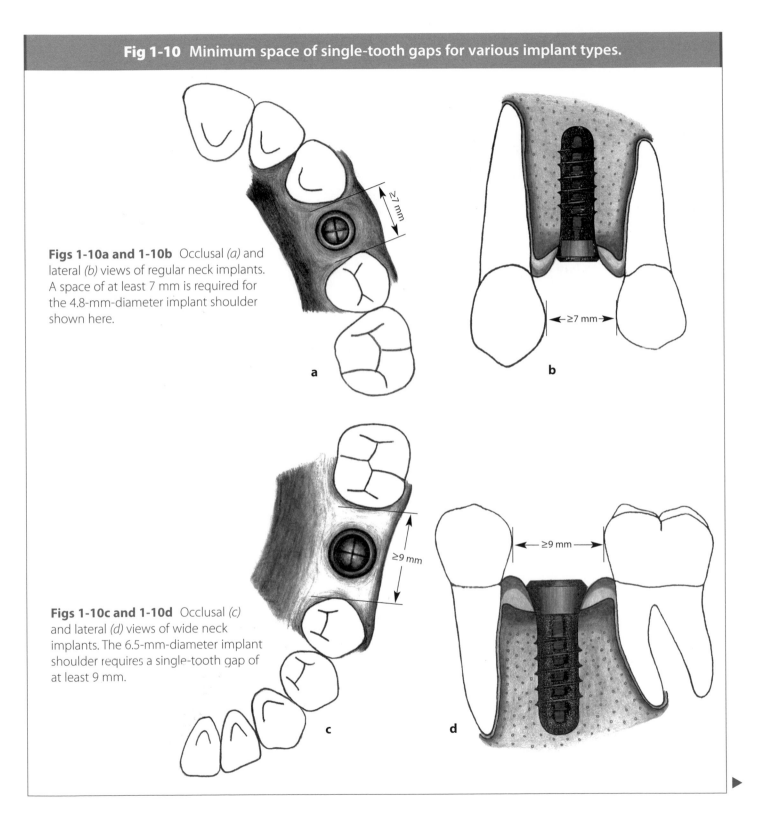

Figs 1-10a and 1-10b Occlusal (a) and lateral (b) views of regular neck implants. A space of at least 7 mm is required for the 4.8-mm-diameter implant shoulder shown here.

≥7 mm

≥7 mm

a

b

Figs 1-10c and 1-10d Occlusal (c) and lateral (d) views of wide neck implants. The 6.5-mm-diameter implant shoulder requires a single-tooth gap of at least 9 mm.

≥9 mm

≥9 mm

c

d

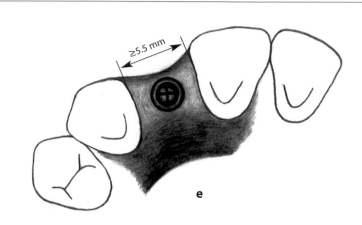

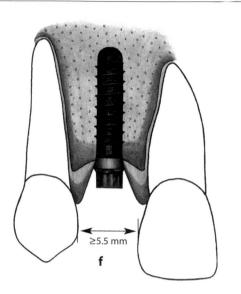

Figs 1-10e and 1-10f Occlusal (e) and lateral (f) views of narrow neck implants. In sites that require narrow neck implants, a minimum of 5.5 mm is needed to accommodate the 3.5-mm-diameter implant shoulder.

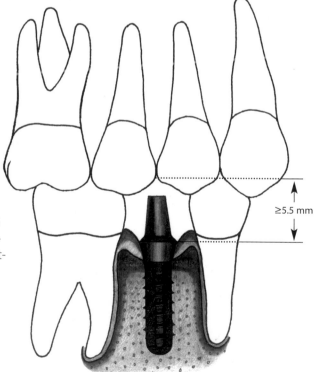

Figs 1-10g A minimum interocclusal distance of 5.5 mm from the implant shoulder to the opposing dentition is necessary to allow the placement of the abutment and crown.

Fig 1-11 Spacing between implants or between implants and teeth.

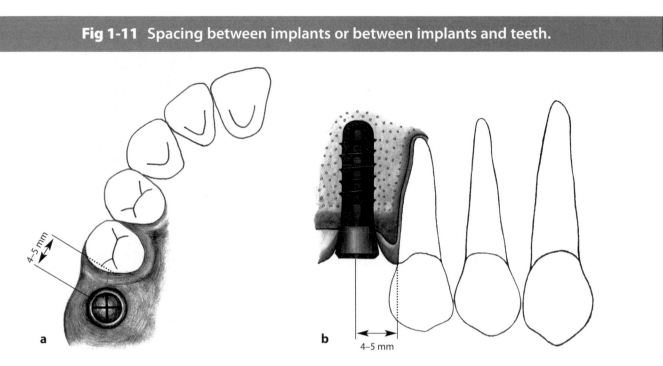

Figs 1-11a and 1-11b Occlusal (a) and lateral (b) views of a regular neck implant placed next to a tooth. A distance of approximately 4 to 5 mm is required between the central axis of the implant and the root surface of the tooth at the alveolar crest.

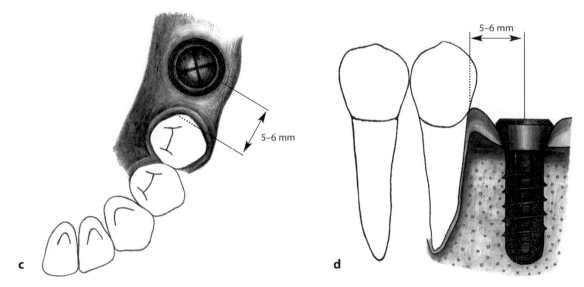

Figs 1-11c and 1-11d Occlusal (c) and lateral (d) views of a wide neck implant placed next to a second premolar. The wide neck implant is positioned approximately 5 to 6 mm from the tooth.

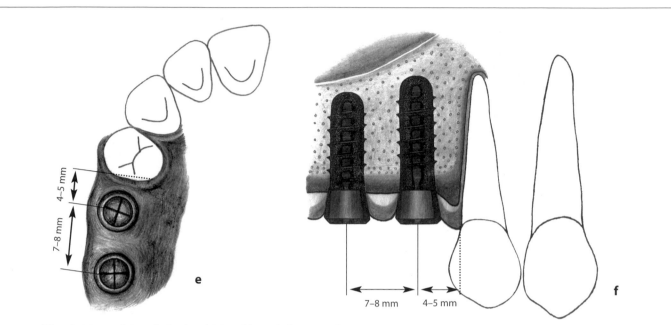

Figs 1-11e and 1-11f Occlusal *(e)* and lateral *(f)* views of regular neck implants. When two regular neck implants are placed side by side in a posterior distal extension situation, the first implant should be positioned 4 to 5 mm from the tooth and the second implant should be positioned 7 to 8 mm from the anterior implant.

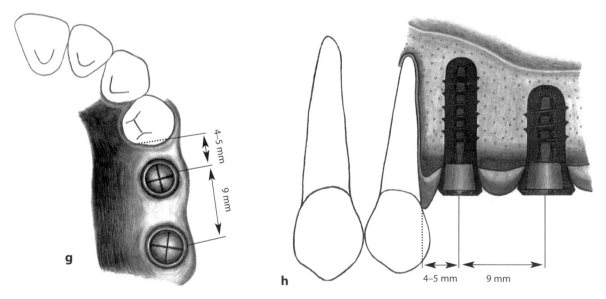

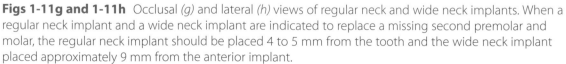

Figs 1-11g and 1-11h Occlusal *(g)* and lateral *(h)* views of regular neck and wide neck implants. When a regular neck implant and a wide neck implant are indicated to replace a missing second premolar and molar, the regular neck implant should be placed 4 to 5 mm from the tooth and the wide neck implant placed approximately 9 mm from the anterior implant.

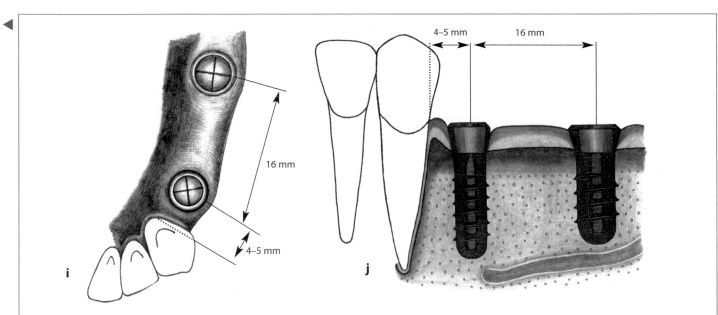

Figs 1-11i and 1-11j Occlusal *(i)* and lateral *(j)* views of implants positioned in the first premolar and first molar sites. In this extended posterior distal extension situation, a regular neck implant and a wide neck implant are indicated as abutments for a three-unit fixed partial denture. The regular neck implant is positioned 4 to 5 mm from the tooth. The wide neck implant is inserted about 16 mm from the anterior implant.

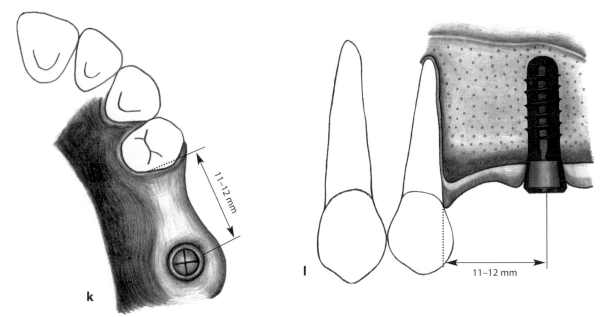

Figs 1-11k and 1-11l Occlusal *(k)* and lateral *(l)* views of a short distal extension situation. A regular neck implant is indicated to restore the missing first molar and serve as a distal abutment to a combined tooth- and implant-supported three-unit fixed partial denture. The implant is positioned 11 to 12 mm from the tooth.

chapter 2

Indications for Each Implant Type

Modern implant systems, such as the Straumann Dental Implant System, offer a variety of different implant types for the various clinical indications of implant therapy. More than 25 years ago, most implant systems offered just one implant type, primarily to treat fully edentulous patients with implant-borne restorations; the standard implant dates back to 1986. Due to the expansion of implant therapy for partially edentulous patients in the late 1980s, the application of implants has steadily increased. In recent years, the single-tooth gap and the distal extension situation have become the two most important indications for implant therapy.

Today, screw-type implants are generally preferred in implant dentistry. Therefore, the diameter of the main implant body with its thread must be differentiated from the diameter of the implant shoulder (other implant systems call it a *platform*). The Straumann Dental Implant System includes three diameters for implant shoulders (ie, regular neck, wide neck, and narrow neck) and three diameters for implant threads (ie, standard, wide body, reduced diameter, and tapered effect).

This chapter presents the author's preferences where these implant types are primarily used.

Fig 2-1   Standard implant.

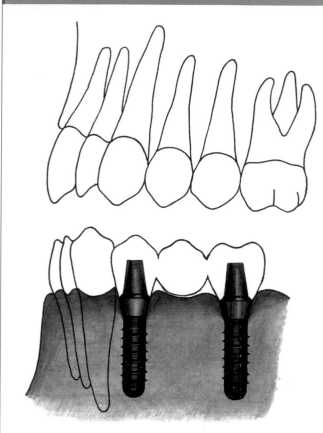

Fig 2-1a Two standard implants are restored with a three-unit fixed partial denture in a mandibular distal extension situation. The implants provide adequate support and function against the opposing dentition.

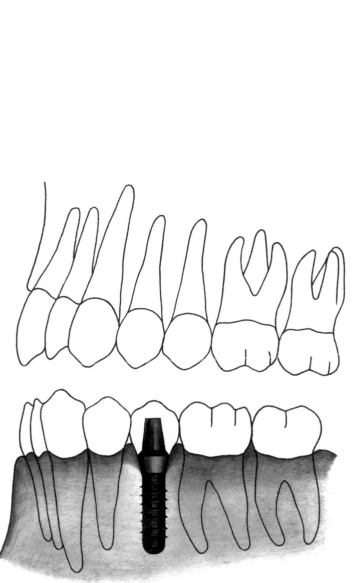

Fig 2-1b For this single-tooth gap, a 12-mm-long standard implant is indicated to replace a missing mandibular second premolar.

Fig 2-2 Standard plus implant.

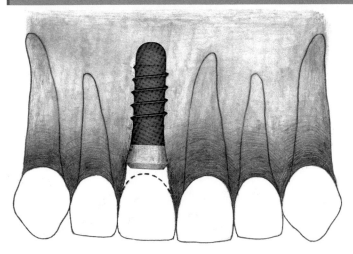

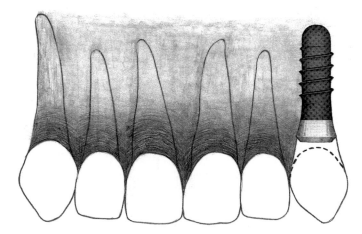

Fig 2-2a In an esthetic restoration involving a single-tooth gap in the anterior region, a standard plus implant is indicated to replace a missing central incisor.

Fig 2-2b A standard plus implant can also be used to replace a maxillary canine in the esthetic zone.

Fig 2-3 Wide body implant.

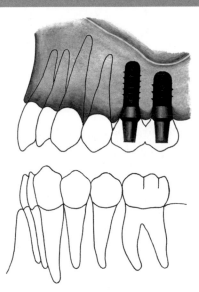

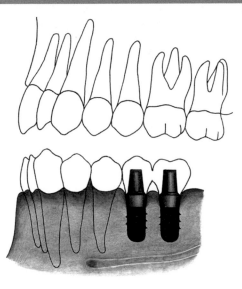

Fig 2-3a Shorter and wider implants are indicated in the posterior maxilla to avoid the maxillary sinus. A standard implant is indicated in the second premolar site, and a wide body implant is indicated in the first molar site.

Fig 2-3b Shorter and wider implants are also indicated in the posterior mandible to avoid the mandibular canal. Two wide body implants can be placed in the first and second molar sites. These implants are restored and, in cases of short 6-mm implants, routinely splinted.

Fig 2-4   Wide neck implant.

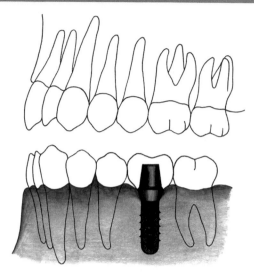

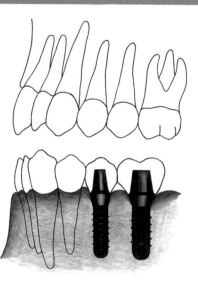

Fig 2-4a A wide neck implant is ideal for a single-tooth gap in the first molar position.

Fig 2-4b In a posterior distal extension situation, a standard implant and a wide neck implant are ideal replacements for a missing second premolar and first molar, respectively.

Fig 2-5   Narrow neck implant.

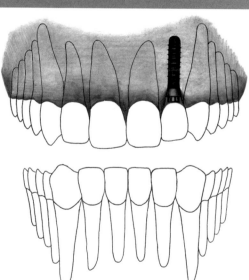

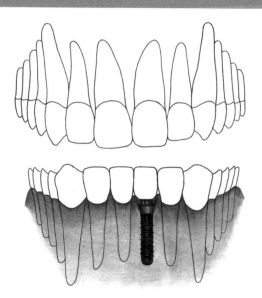

Fig 2-5a A narrow neck implant is indicated to replace a missing lateral incisor where the single-tooth gap offers limited space.

Fig 2-5b Another indication for a narrow neck implant is to replace missing mandibular incisors where available tooth space is likewise restricted.

Fig 2-6 Reduced-diameter implant.

Fig 2-6 For situations in which the posterior distal extension has inadequate alveolar ridge width, reduced-diameter implants can be used in premolar sites, whereas a standard implant can be placed in the first molar position. Splinting of the crowns is recommended when implants of reduced diameter are used.

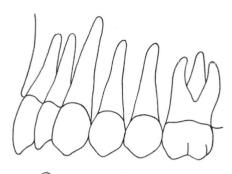
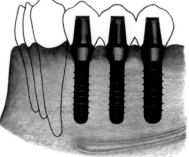

Fig 2-7 Tapered effect implant.

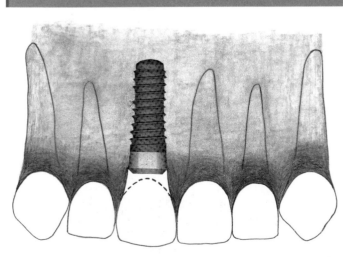
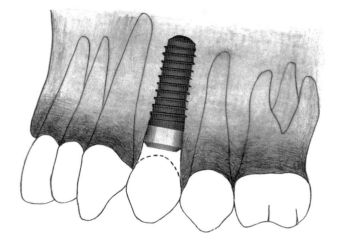

Fig 2-7a For a single-tooth gap following an extraction in the anterior maxilla, a tapered effect implant is indicated to replace a missing central incisor.

Fig 2-7b In the extraction socket of a first premolar, a tapered effect implant can also be indicated for early implant placement.

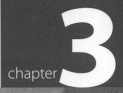
Surgical Procedures in Standard Nonesthetic Sites

The majority of surgical implant procedures are performed in nonesthetic sites, most often for implant placement in premolar and molar sites in the mandible and maxilla. The primary objective of therapy in these sites is to reestablish masticatory function with a fixed restoration.

This chapter deals with implant surgery in standard sites without bone deficiencies. The clinical situations represent a simple, straightforward level of difficulty. Details of flap elevation, implant site preparation, implant insertion, and soft tissue suturing using a nonsubmerged approach are presented. The surgical steps illustrate the most important indication in posterior sites, the distal extension situation.

Fig 3-1 **Flap elevation in a mandibular distal extension situation.**

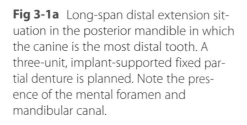

Fig 3-1a Long-span distal extension situation in the posterior mandible in which the canine is the most distal tooth. A three-unit, implant-supported fixed partial denture is planned. Note the presence of the mental foramen and mandibular canal.

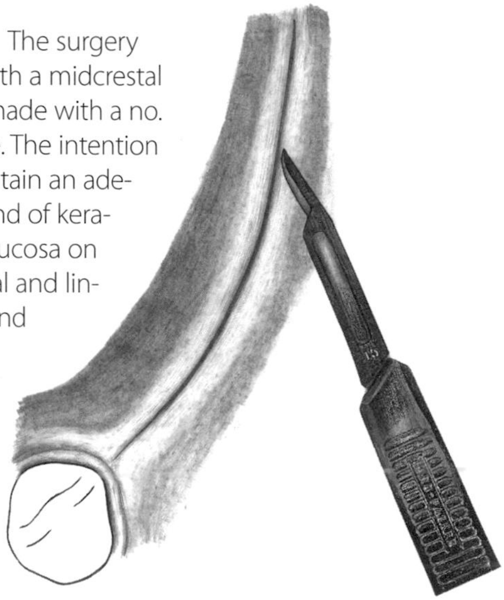

Fig 3-1b The surgery begins with a midcrestal incision made with a no. 15c blade. The intention is to maintain an adequate band of keratinized mucosa on the buccal and lingual wound margins.

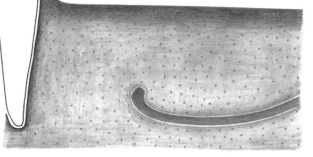

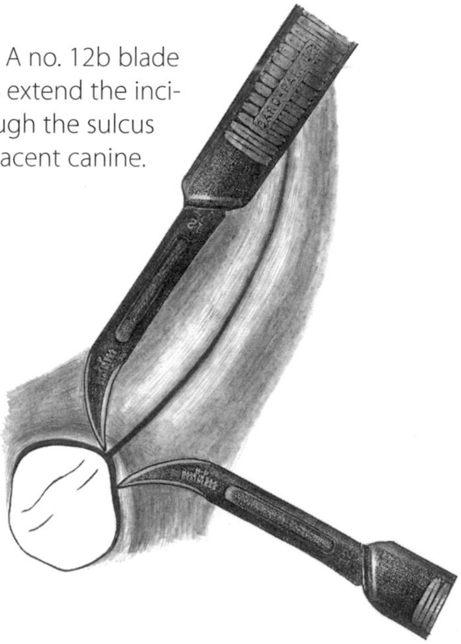

Fig 3-1c A no. 12b blade is used to extend the incision through the sulcus of the adjacent canine.

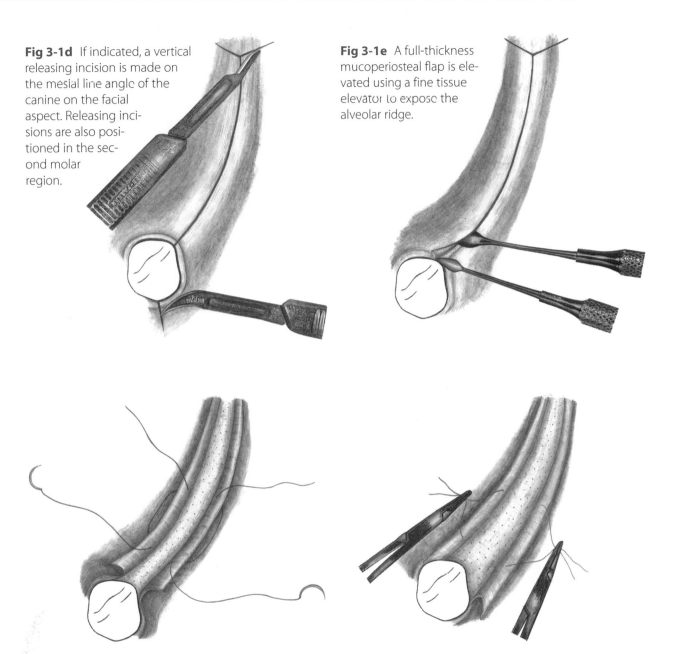

Fig 3-1d If indicated, a vertical releasing incision is made on the mesial line angle of the canine on the facial aspect. Releasing incisions are also positioned in the second molar region.

Fig 3-1e A full-thickness mucoperiosteal flap is elevated using a fine tissue elevator to expose the alveolar ridge.

Fig 3-1f Retraction mattress sutures are attached to the buccal and lingual flaps to allow sufficient access to the implant sites.

Fig 3-1g The retraction sutures are attached to hemostats to keep the flaps opened and in place.

Fig 3-2   Implant site preparation in a mandibular distal extension situation.

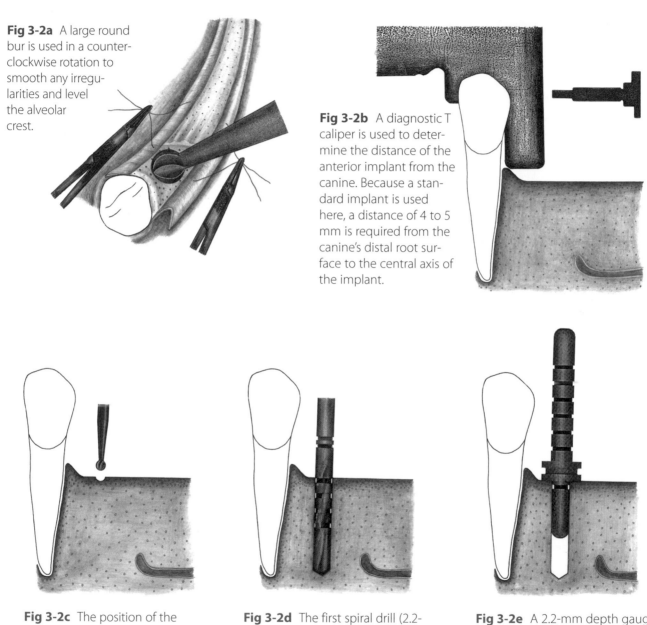

Fig 3-2a A large round bur is used in a counterclockwise rotation to smooth any irregularities and level the alveolar crest.

Fig 3-2b A diagnostic T caliper is used to determine the distance of the anterior implant from the canine. Because a standard implant is used here, a distance of 4 to 5 mm is required from the canine's distal root surface to the central axis of the implant.

Fig 3-2c The position of the anterior implant is marked with a small round bur.

Fig 3-2d The first spiral drill (2.2-mm diameter) is easily positioned, and the site is prepared to a depth of 12 mm.

Fig 3-2e A 2.2-mm depth gauge with a 5-mm platform ring is inserted to check the correct distance from the adjacent canine.

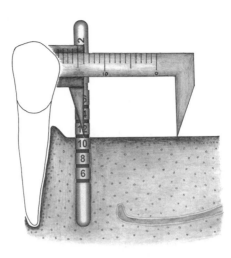

Fig 3-2f A pair of calipers is used to locate the position of the posterior implant by measuring a distance of 14 mm from the anterior implant.

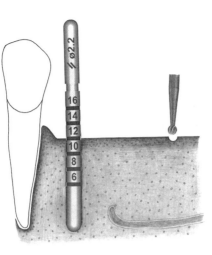

Fig 3-2g The same small round bur is used to mark the second implant site.

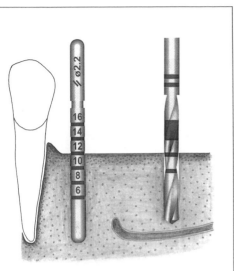

Fig 3-2h The 2.2-mm-diameter spiral drill prepares the site to a depth of 8 mm to avoid the mandibular canal.

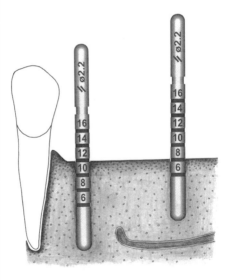

Fig 3-2i The 2.2-mm guide pins are inserted into the site preparations to check their positions and the parallelism of their axes.

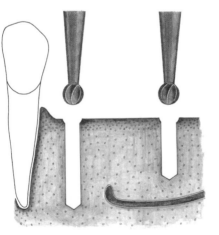

Fig 3-2j The openings of the implant site preparations are enlarged using a larger round bur.

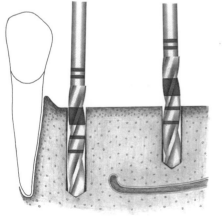

Fig 3-2k The 2.8-mm-diameter spiral drill is inserted to the predetermined depth at each implant site.

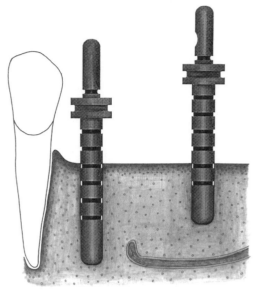

Fig 3-2l The sink depths and parallel axes for the implant preparations are examined with the 2.8-mm-diameter depth gauges in situ.

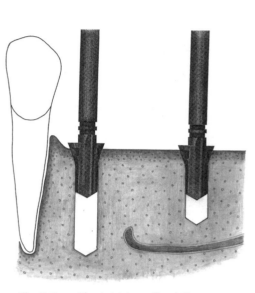

Fig 3-2m The initial profile drills are now used to prepare the coronal aspect of the implant site preparations.

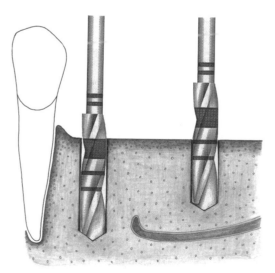

Fig 3-2n Drilling continues with the use of the 3.5-mm-diameter spiral drills prepared to the correct depths.

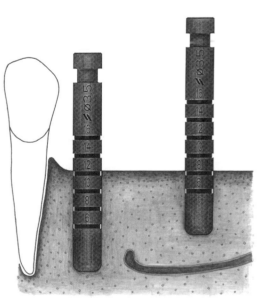

Fig 3-2o The sink depths and parallel axes of the preparation sites are again examined with the 3.5-mm depth gauges.

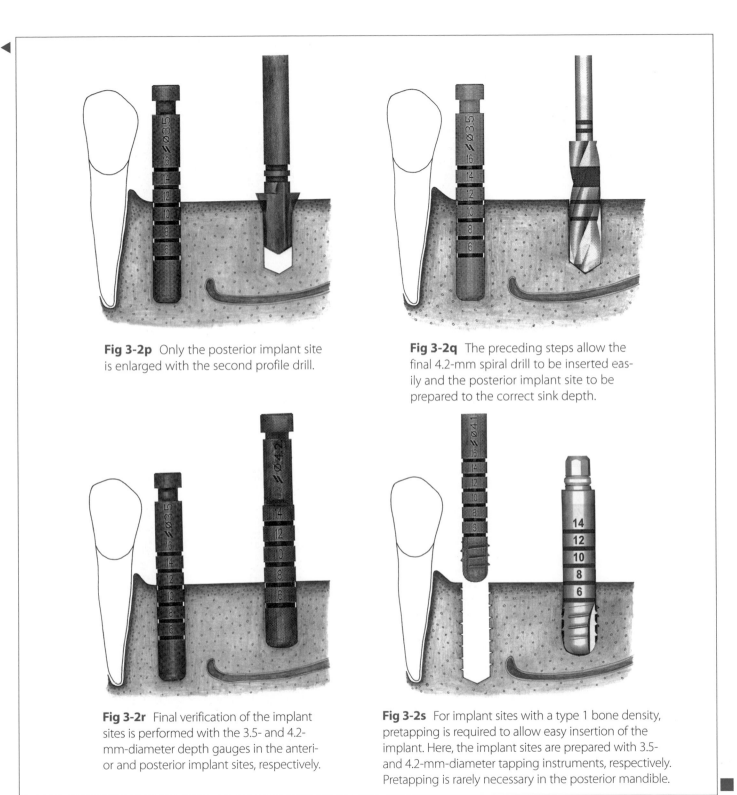

Fig 3-2p Only the posterior implant site is enlarged with the second profile drill.

Fig 3-2q The preceding steps allow the final 4.2-mm spiral drill to be inserted easily and the posterior implant site to be prepared to the correct sink depth.

Fig 3-2r Final verification of the implant sites is performed with the 3.5- and 4.2-mm-diameter depth gauges in the anterior and posterior implant sites, respectively.

Fig 3-2s For implant sites with a type 1 bone density, pretapping is required to allow easy insertion of the implant. Here, the implant sites are prepared with 3.5- and 4.2-mm-diameter tapping instruments, respectively. Pretapping is rarely necessary in the posterior mandible.

Fig 3-3 Implant placement in a mandibular distal extension situation.

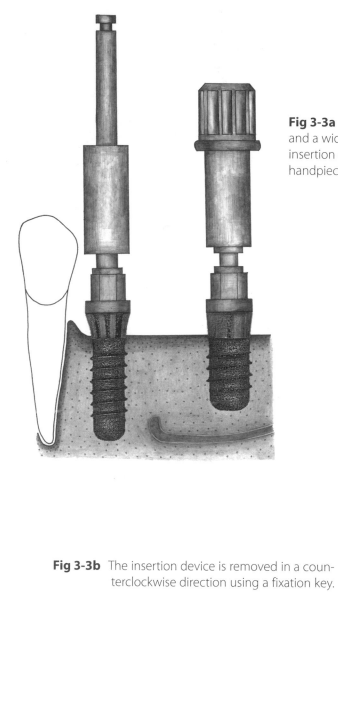

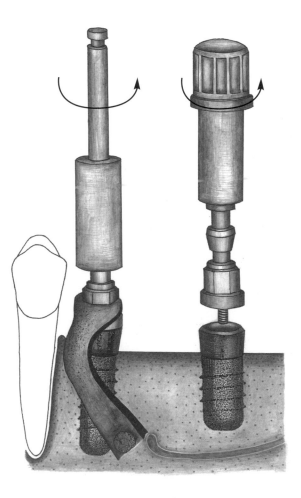

Fig 3-3a A standard implant is inserted in the anterior site and a wide body implant is inserted in the posterior site. The insertion device can be attached to a low-speed contra-angle handpiece (15 rpm) *(left)* or to a hand ratchet device *(right)*.

Fig 3-3b The insertion device is removed in a counterclockwise direction using a fixation key.

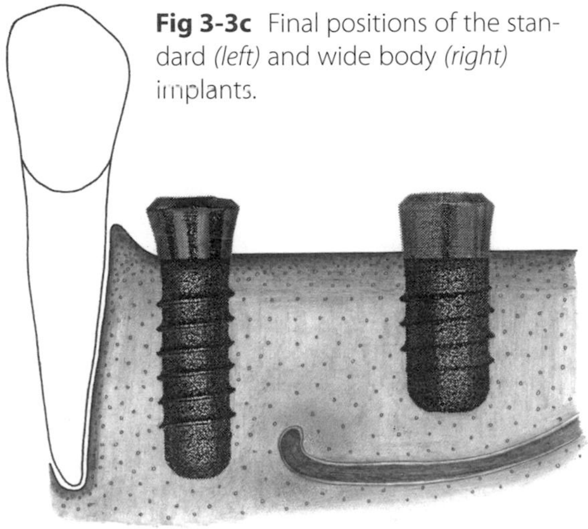

Fig 3-3c Final positions of the standard *(left)* and wide body *(right)* implants.

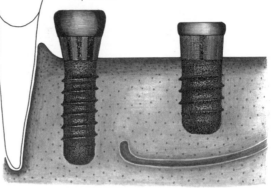

Fig 3-3d Healing caps for the mesial implant (3 mm) and the distal implant (1.5 mm) are attached to cover the implants.

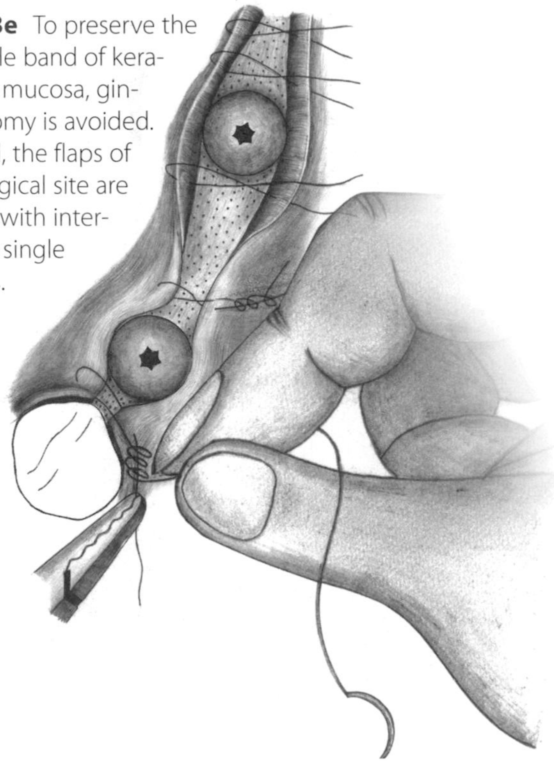

Fig 3-3e To preserve the available band of keratinized mucosa, gingivectomy is avoided. Instead, the flaps of the surgical site are closed with interrupted single sutures.

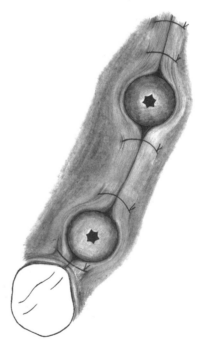

Fig 3-3f Complete closure following suturing. In standard posterior sites without bone deficiency, a nonsubmerged healing modality is routinely used. Soft tissue healing requires a period of 10 to 14 days.

Fig 3-4 Soft tissue suturing of a mandibular distal extension situation with one implant.

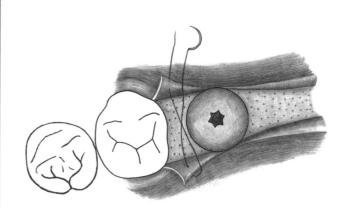

Fig 3-4a Occlusal view following placement of a wide neck implant in the mandibular first molar site. Closure of the flaps begins with the mesial papilla.

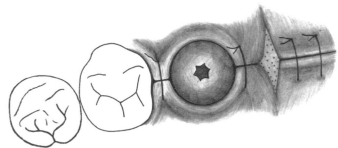

Fig 3-4b Once the mesial papilla is secured, relieving incisions are made approximately 3 mm distal to the implant to ensure a tension-free closure and obtain an adequate band of keratinized mucosa surrounding the implant.

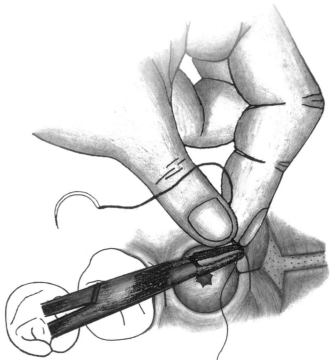

Fig 3-4c The buccal and lingual wound margins are rotated in slightly and sutured.

Fig 3-4d The remaining surgical site is closed with interrupted single sutures. The slight exposure of the bone distal to the implant site will heal by granulation.

Fig 3-5 Soft tissue suturing of two implants with adequate keratinized mucosa.

Fig 3-5a In sites with adequate keratinized mucosa surrounding two adjacent implants, a modified procedure is used to achieve flap closure. The mesial papilla is closed first with an interrupted single suture. Two Palacci incisions are made into the keratinized wound margin with a new no. 15c blade.

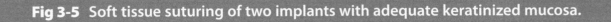

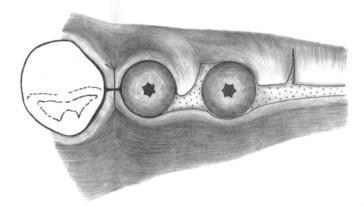

Fig 3-5b The newly created Palacci flaps are rotated in to provide a more favorable proximal soft tissue adaptation and closure.

Fig 3-5c The flaps are approximated and closed with several interrupted single sutures.

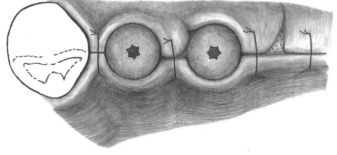

Fig 3-6 Alternative method for soft tissue suturing of two implants with adequate keratinized mucosa.

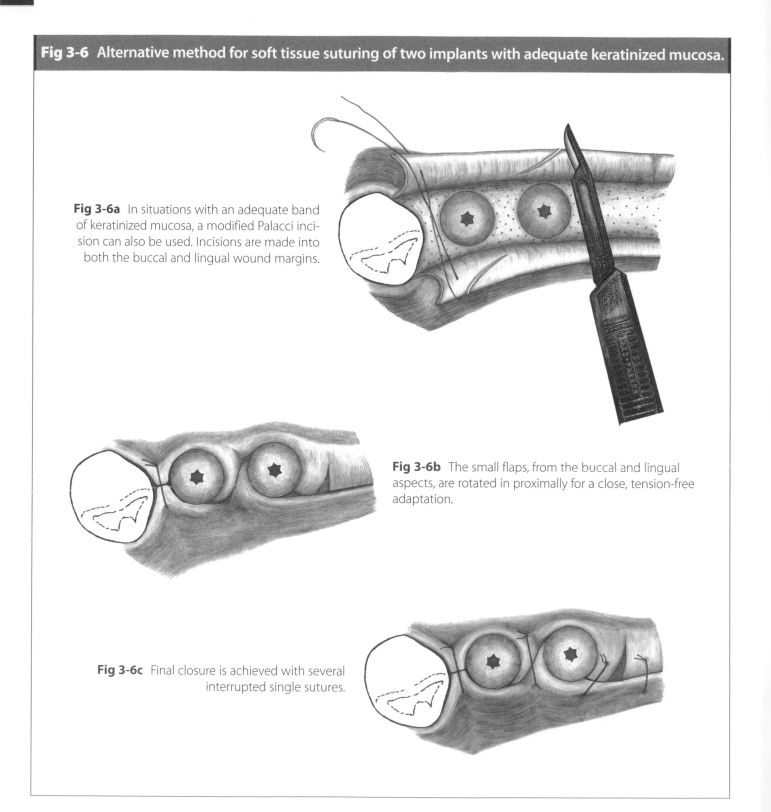

Fig 3-6a In situations with an adequate band of keratinized mucosa, a modified Palacci incision can also be used. Incisions are made into both the buccal and lingual wound margins.

Fig 3-6b The small flaps, from the buccal and lingual aspects, are rotated in proximally for a close, tension-free adaptation.

Fig 3-6c Final closure is achieved with several interrupted single sutures.

Fig 3-7 Soft tissue suturing of two implants with inadequate keratinized mucosa in the mandible.

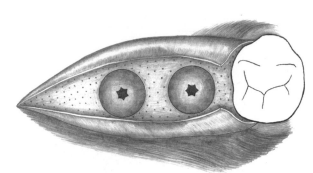

Fig 3-7a For cases in which minimal keratinized mucosa surrounds two adjacent implants, adjunctive grafting procedures may be necessary for better management of the soft tissues.

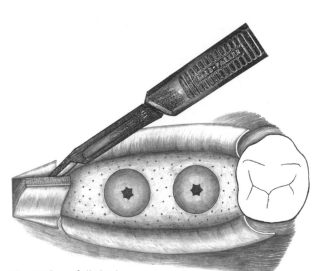

Fig 3-7b A full-thickness mucosal graft is harvested from the retromolar area.

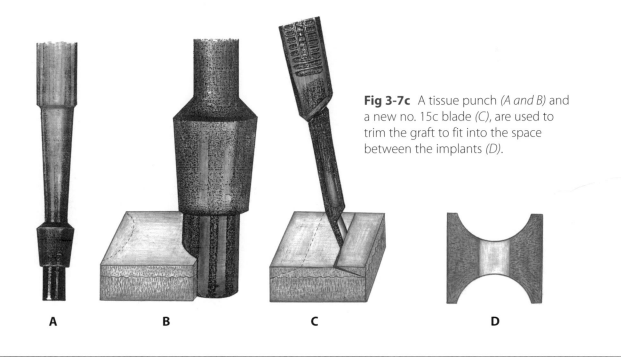

Fig 3-7c A tissue punch (*A and B*) and a new no. 15c blade (*C*), are used to trim the graft to fit into the space between the implants (*D*).

A   B   C   D

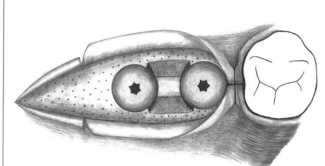

Fig 3-7d The graft is placed in the interproximal space between the implants. Meanwhile, the mesial papilla is sutured.

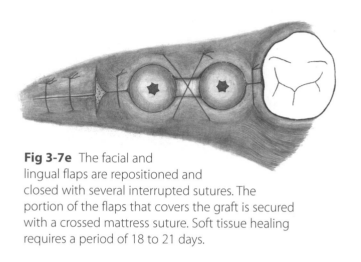

Fig 3-7e The facial and lingual flaps are repositioned and closed with several interrupted sutures. The portion of the flaps that covers the graft is secured with a crossed mattress suture. Soft tissue healing requires a period of 18 to 21 days.

Fig 3-8   **Soft tissue suturing of two implants with inadequate keratinized mucosa in the maxilla.**

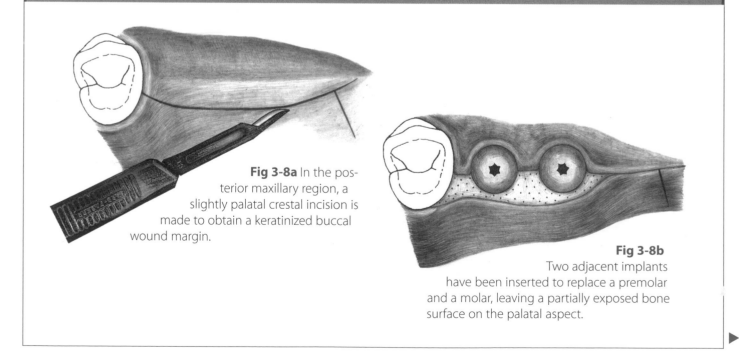

Fig 3-8a In the posterior maxillary region, a slightly palatal crestal incision is made to obtain a keratinized buccal wound margin.

Fig 3-8b Two adjacent implants have been inserted to replace a premolar and a molar, leaving a partially exposed bone surface on the palatal aspect.

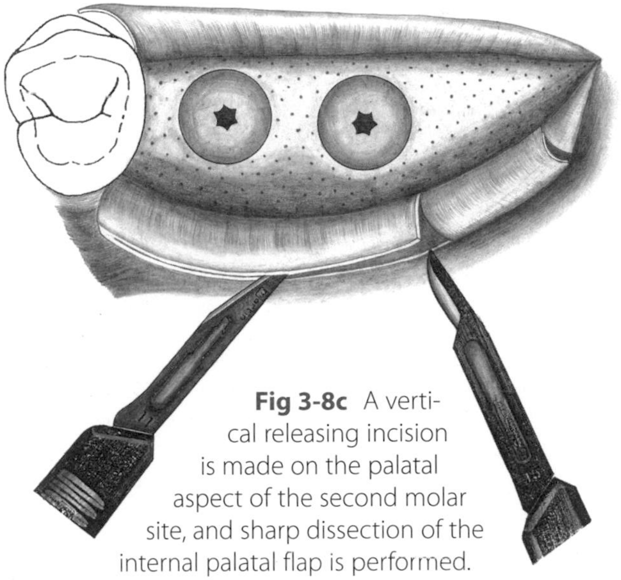

Fig 3-8c A vertical releasing incision is made on the palatal aspect of the second molar site, and sharp dissection of the internal palatal flap is performed.

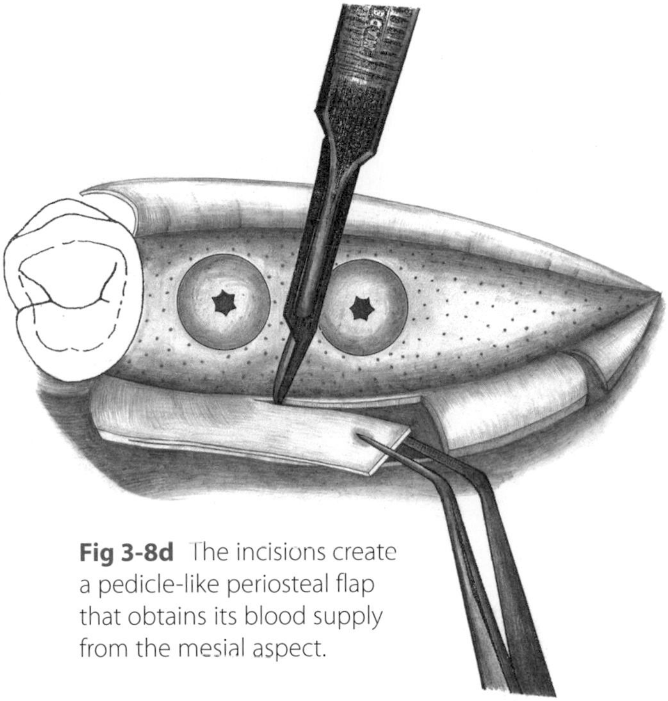

Fig 3-8d The incisions create a pedicle-like periosteal flap that obtains its blood supply from the mesial aspect.

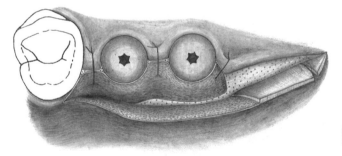

Fig 3-8e The pedicle flap is rotated toward the exposed palatal crest around the implants and sutured into place.

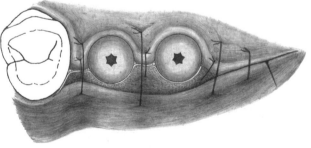

Fig 3-8f Final closure of the main palatal flap partially covering the rotated pedicle flap is performed with large interrupted single sutures. Soft tissue healing by granulation will require 21 to 28 days to achieve full keratinization of the palatal mucosa.

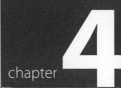

chapter 4

Surgical Procedures in Standard Esthetic Sites

Implant therapy in esthetic sites is challenging for clinicians and represents an advanced level of difficulty. The extension of the esthetic zone in the maxilla depends on the patient's smile line and can include the premolars or even the first molars.

This chapters presents the basic surgical procedures in two standard esthetic sites in the anterior maxilla without bone deficiencies. This clinical situation is not frequently seen today, since implants are often placed in the anterior maxilla in sites with local bone defects (eg, following tooth extraction). Nevertheless, the basic principles governing flap elevation, correct three-dimensional implant positioning, and soft tissue suturing are valid for esthetic sites in general and apply for implant placement with simultaneous bone augmentation procedures as well, which are presented in chapter 5.

Fig 4-1 **Flap elevation in a maxillary central incisor site.**

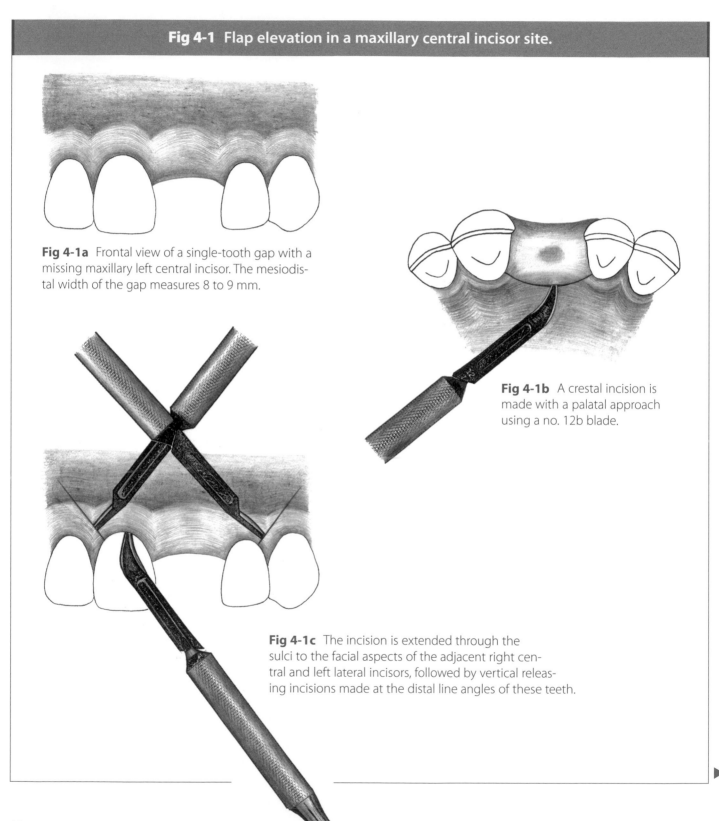

Fig 4-1a Frontal view of a single-tooth gap with a missing maxillary left central incisor. The mesiodistal width of the gap measures 8 to 9 mm.

Fig 4-1b A crestal incision is made with a palatal approach using a no. 12b blade.

Fig 4-1c The incision is extended through the sulci to the facial aspects of the adjacent right central and left lateral incisors, followed by vertical releasing incisions made at the distal line angles of these teeth.

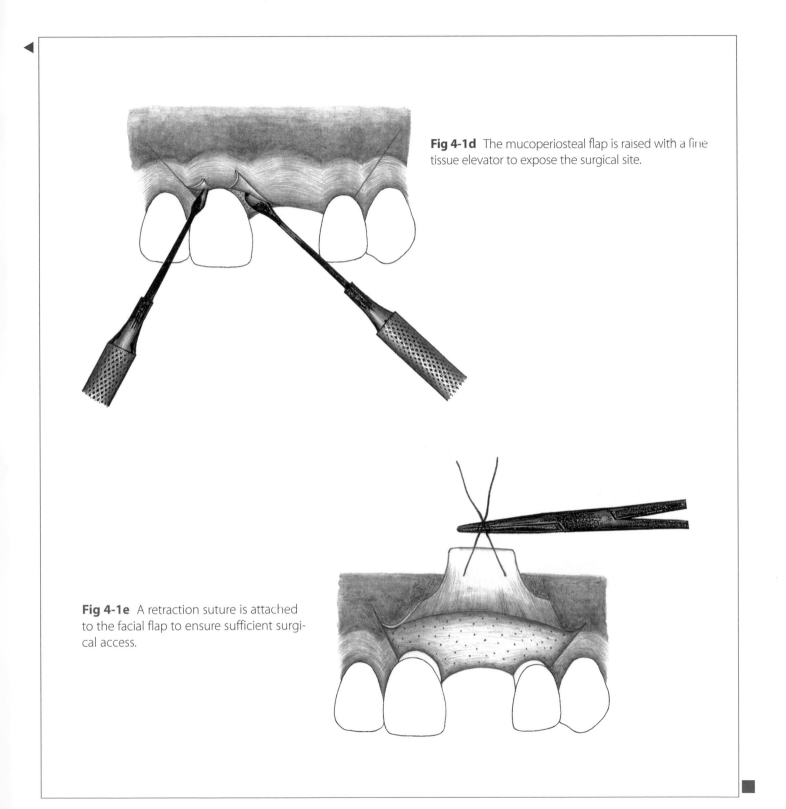

Fig 4-1d The mucoperiosteal flap is raised with a fine tissue elevator to expose the surgical site.

Fig 4-1e A retraction suture is attached to the facial flap to ensure sufficient surgical access.

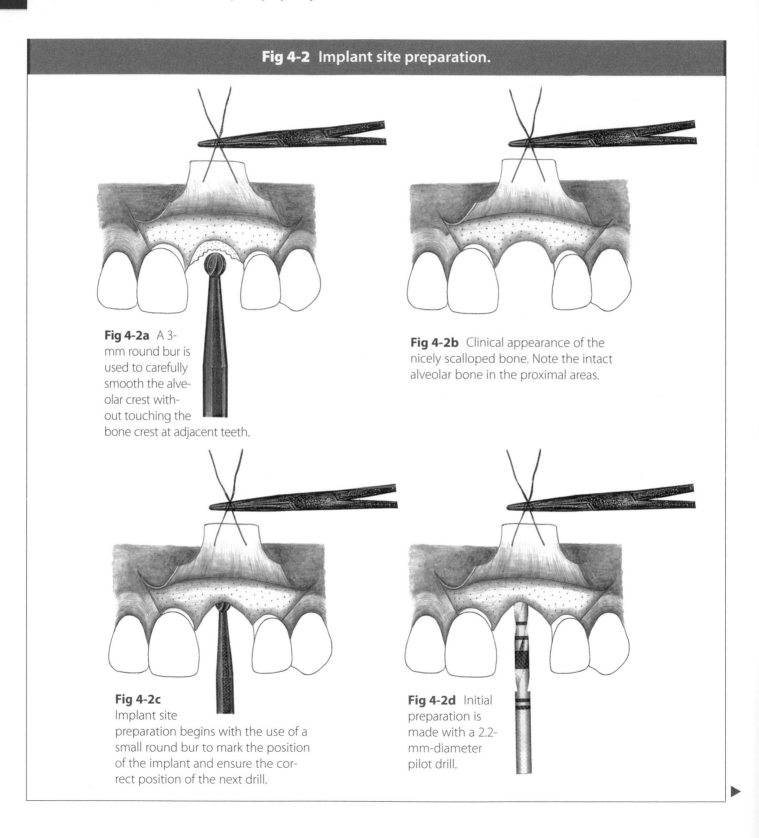

Fig 4-2 Implant site preparation.

Fig 4-2a A 3-mm round bur is used to carefully smooth the alveolar crest without touching the bone crest at adjacent teeth.

Fig 4-2b Clinical appearance of the nicely scalloped bone. Note the intact alveolar bone in the proximal areas.

Fig 4-2c Implant site preparation begins with the use of a small round bur to mark the position of the implant and ensure the correct position of the next drill.

Fig 4-2d Initial preparation is made with a 2.2-mm-diameter pilot drill.

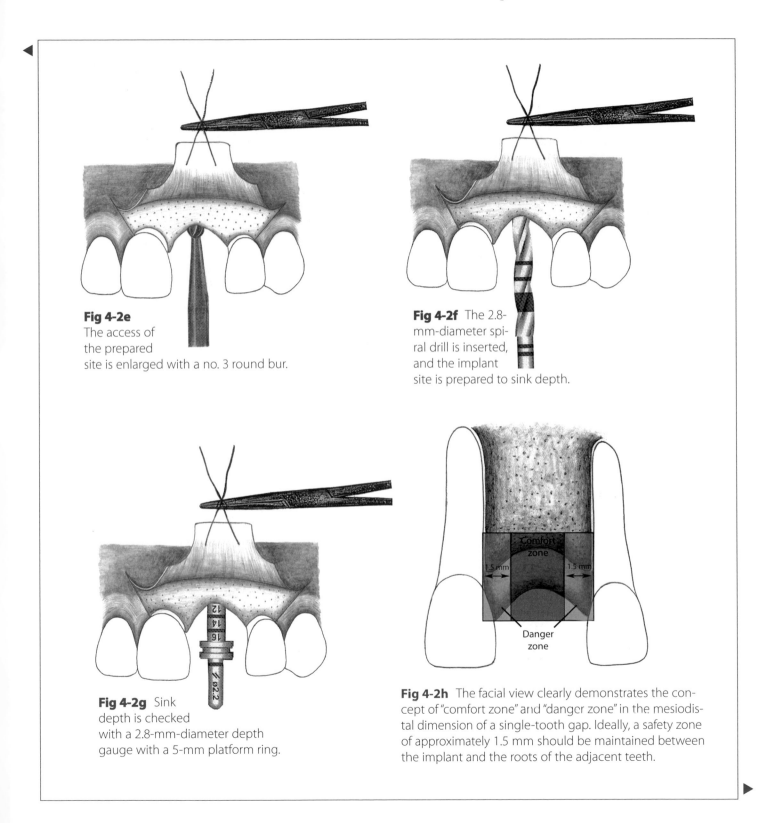

Fig 4-2e
The access of
the prepared
site is enlarged with a no. 3 round bur.

Fig 4-2f The 2.8-
mm-diameter spi-
ral drill is inserted,
and the implant
site is prepared to sink depth.

Fig 4-2g Sink
depth is checked
with a 2.8-mm-diameter depth
gauge with a 5-mm platform ring.

Fig 4-2h The facial view clearly demonstrates the concept of "comfort zone" and "danger zone" in the mesiodistal dimension of a single-tooth gap. Ideally, a safety zone
of approximately 1.5 mm should be maintained between
the implant and the roots of the adjacent teeth.

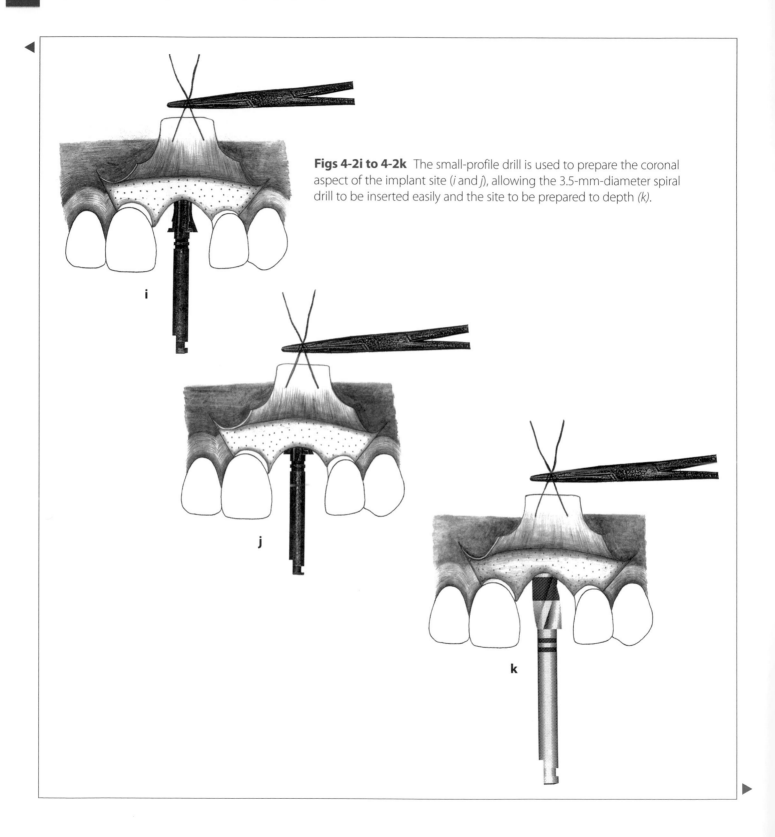

Figs 4-2i to 4-2k The small-profile drill is used to prepare the coronal aspect of the implant site (*i* and *j*), allowing the 3.5-mm-diameter spiral drill to be inserted easily and the site to be prepared to depth (*k*).

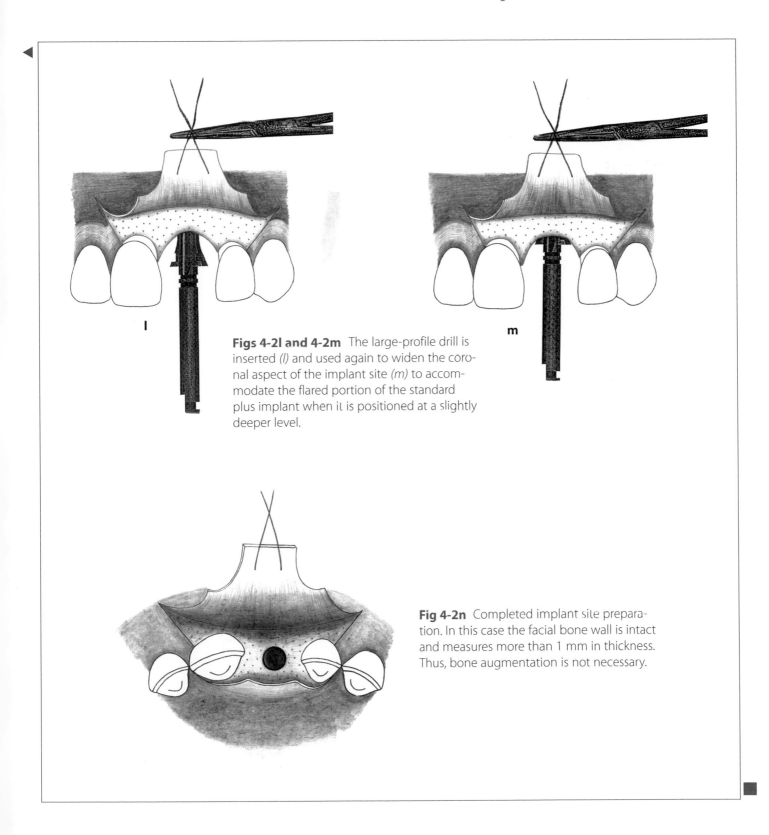

Figs 4-2l and 4-2m The large-profile drill is inserted (l) and used again to widen the coronal aspect of the implant site (m) to accommodate the flared portion of the standard plus implant when it is positioned at a slightly deeper level.

Fig 4-2n Completed implant site preparation. In this case the facial bone wall is intact and measures more than 1 mm in thickness. Thus, bone augmentation is not necessary.

Fig 4-3 Implant placement with correct three-dimensional positioning.

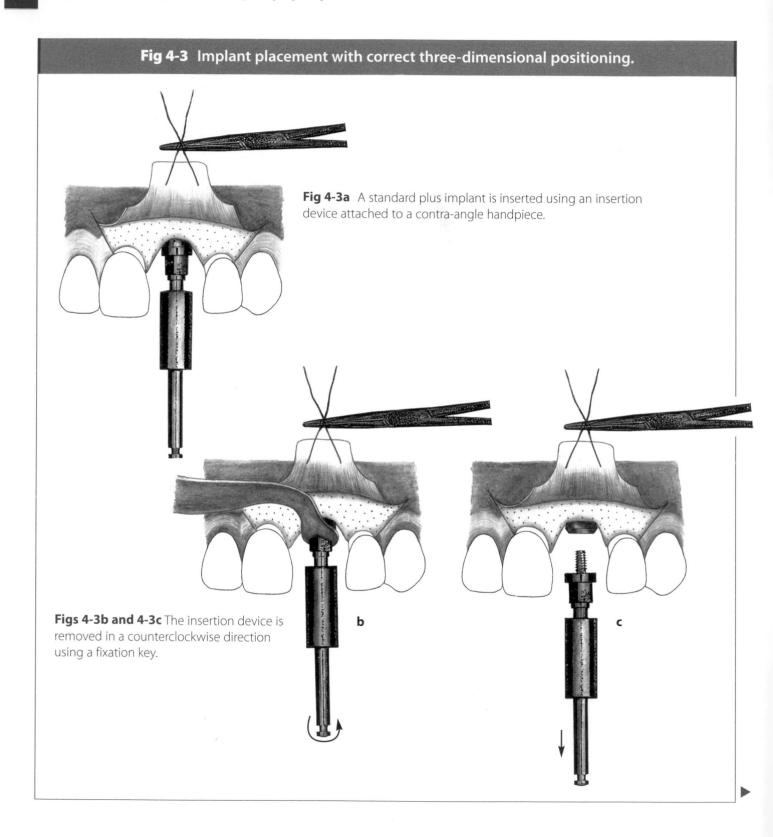

Fig 4-3a A standard plus implant is inserted using an insertion device attached to a contra-angle handpiece.

Figs 4-3b and 4-3c The insertion device is removed in a counterclockwise direction using a fixation key.

b

c

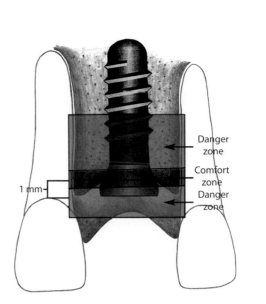

Fig 4-3d Site analysis with the implant in place. The frontal view demonstrates the correct vertical positioning of the implant with respect to the periodontal probe. Ideally, the implant shoulder should be positioned approximately 1 mm apical to the cementoenamel junction (CEJ) of the adjacent contralateral tooth.

Fig 4-3e Facial view of the final coronoapical positioning of the implant. The shoulder of the implant should be placed within the limited comfort zone approximately 1 mm apical to the CEJ of the contralateral incisor.

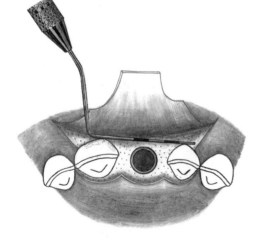

Fig 4-3f Occlusally, the periodontal probe at the CEJ of the adjacent teeth confirms good orofacial positioning of the implant. The anterior margin of the implant shoulder should be positioned 1 mm palatal to the probe.

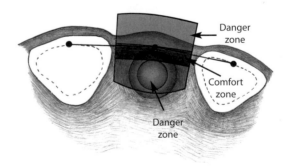

Fig 4-3g From the occlusal view, an imaginary line can be drawn across the facial aspect of the adjacent teeth. Ideally, the shoulder of the implant should be located in the comfort zone, approximately 1.0 to 1.5 mm palatal to this line.

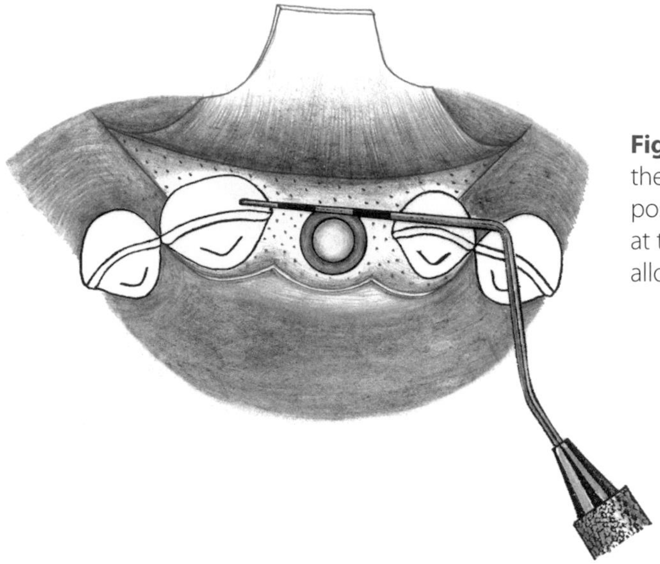

Fig 4-3h A pin is inserted into the implant to indicate the prosthetic axis. The implant demonstrates excellent positioning with respect to the periodontal probe placed at the incisal edges of the adjacent teeth, which will allow for easy transocclusal screw retention of the crown.

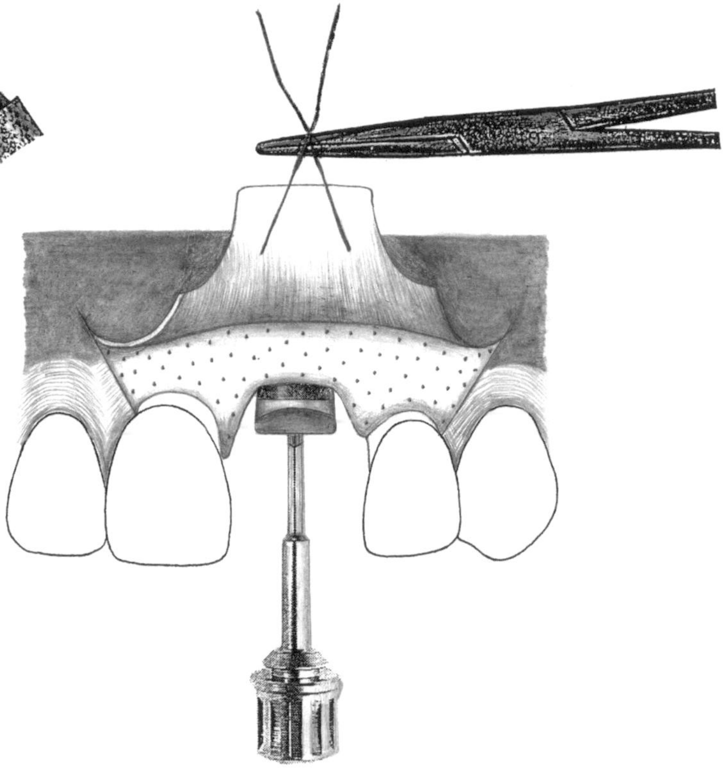

Fig 4-3i A short healing cap with a buccal bevel is inserted.

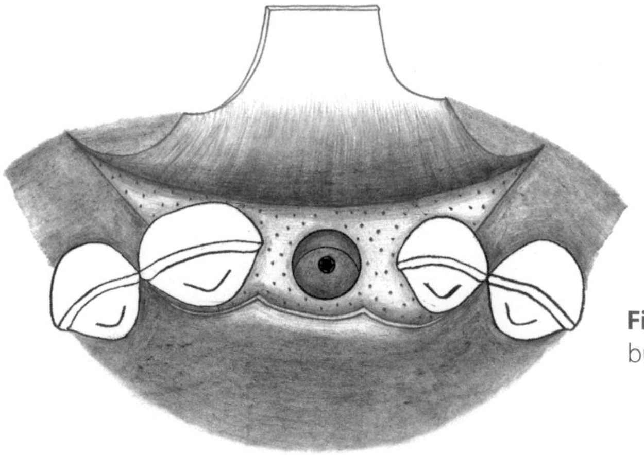

Fig 4-3j Occlusal view of the healing cap with the buccal bevel.

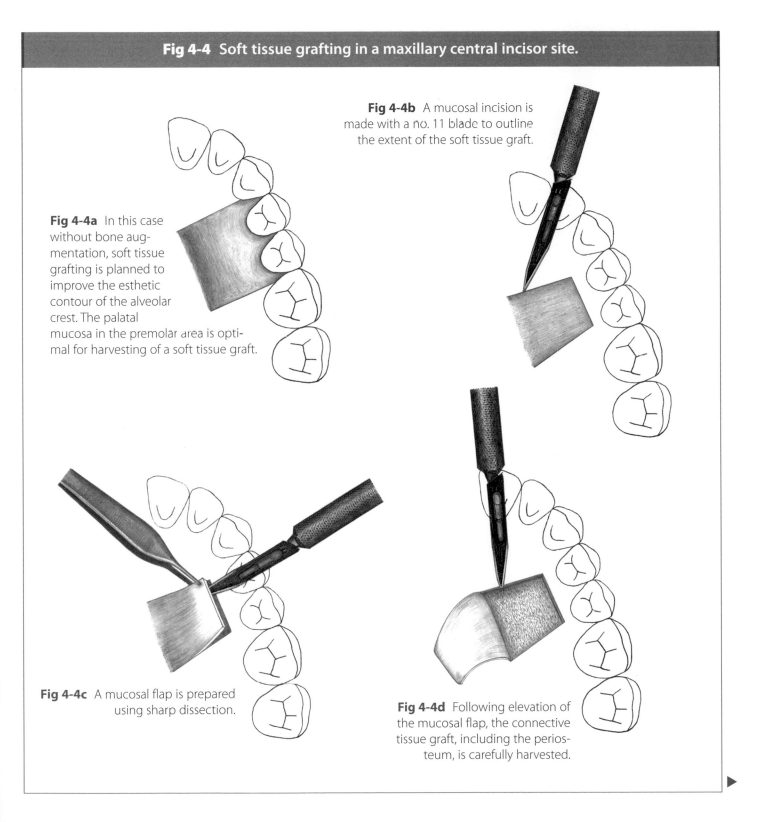

Fig 4-4 Soft tissue grafting in a maxillary central incisor site.

Fig 4-4a In this case without bone augmentation, soft tissue grafting is planned to improve the esthetic contour of the alveolar crest. The palatal mucosa in the premolar area is optimal for harvesting of a soft tissue graft.

Fig 4-4b A mucosal incision is made with a no. 11 blade to outline the extent of the soft tissue graft.

Fig 4-4c A mucosal flap is prepared using sharp dissection.

Fig 4-4d Following elevation of the mucosal flap, the connective tissue graft, including the periosteum, is carefully harvested.

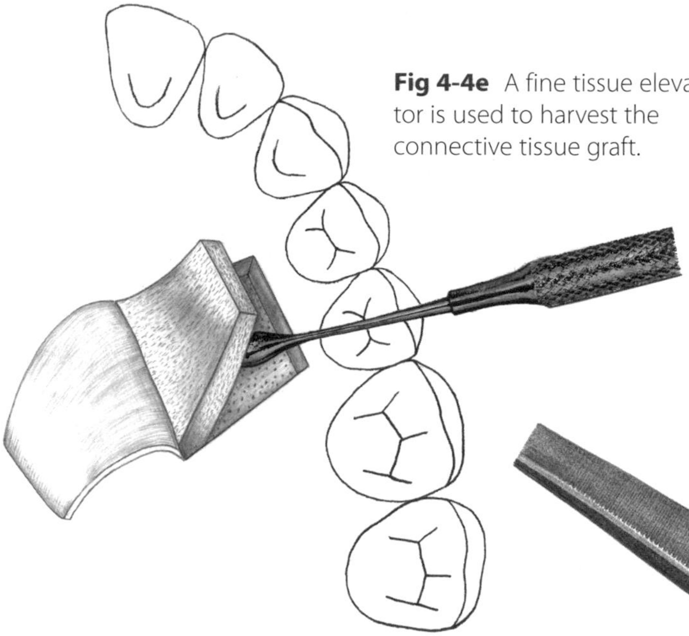

Fig 4-4e A fine tissue eleva-tor is used to harvest the connective tissue graft.

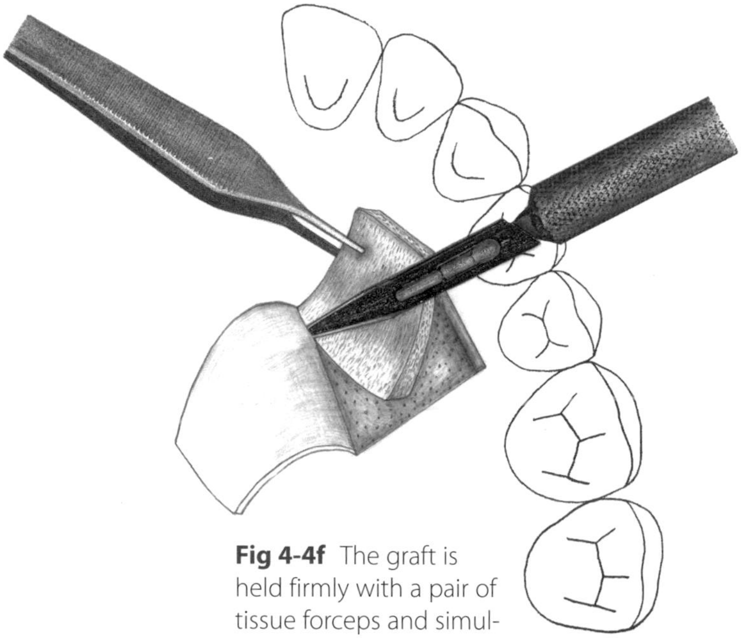

Fig 4-4f The graft is held firmly with a pair of tissue forceps and simul-taneously removed with the no. 11 blade.

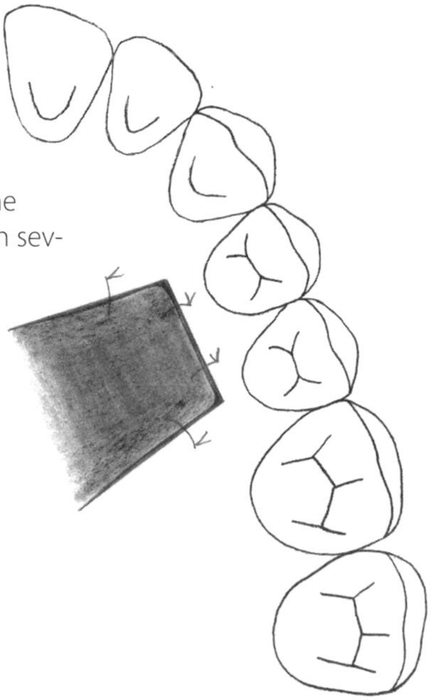

Fig 4-4g The flap of the donor site is closed with sev-eral interrupted single sutures.

Fig 4-5 Wound closure in a maxillary central incisor site.

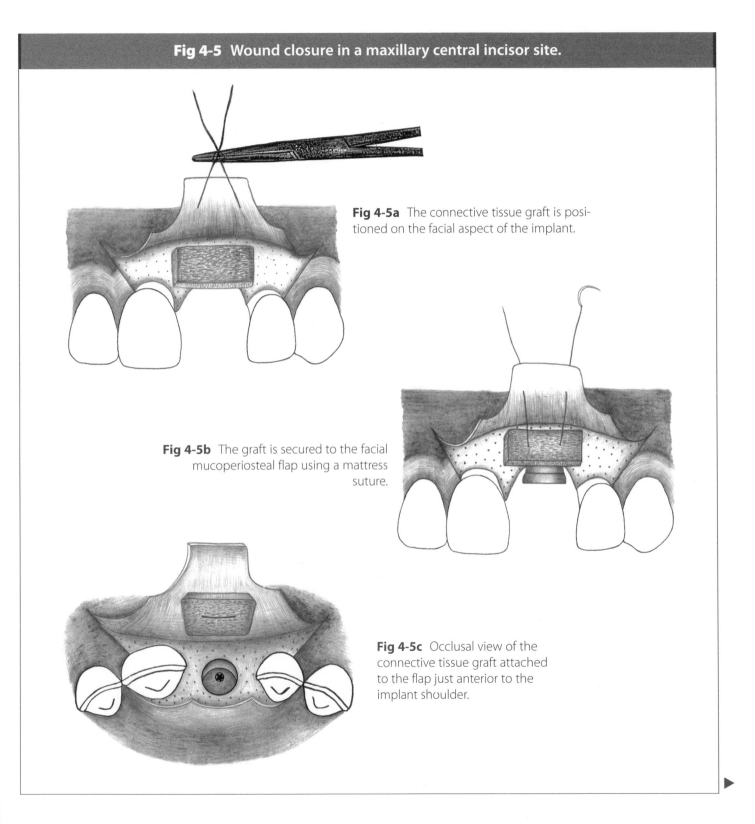

Fig 4-5a The connective tissue graft is positioned on the facial aspect of the implant.

Fig 4-5b The graft is secured to the facial mucoperiosteal flap using a mattress suture.

Fig 4-5c Occlusal view of the connective tissue graft attached to the flap just anterior to the implant shoulder.

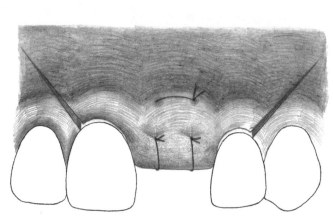

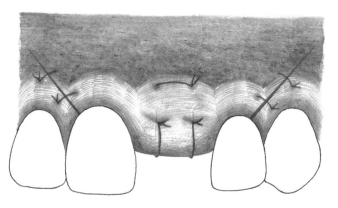

Fig 4-5d Two single crestal sutures are attached, and the flap is repositioned and closed to complete the surgery. Nonresorbable monofilament 5-0 suture material is preferred.

Fig 4-5e The releasing incisions are closed with several interrupted single sutures of fine 6-0 suture material. As in most esthetic sites, submerged healing is preferred.

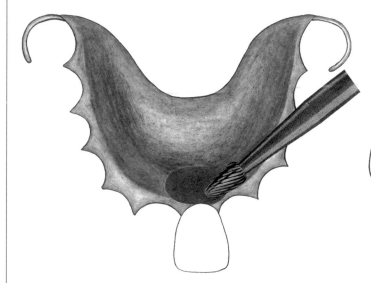

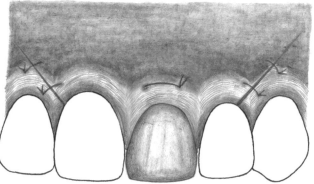

Fig 4-5g Frontal view showing the provisional removable partial denture adjusted and positioned passively over the surgical site.

Fig 4-5f Before the patient is sent home, the provisional removable partial denture is trimmed using an acrylic bur to prevent any excessive pressure on the surgical site during the healing phase.

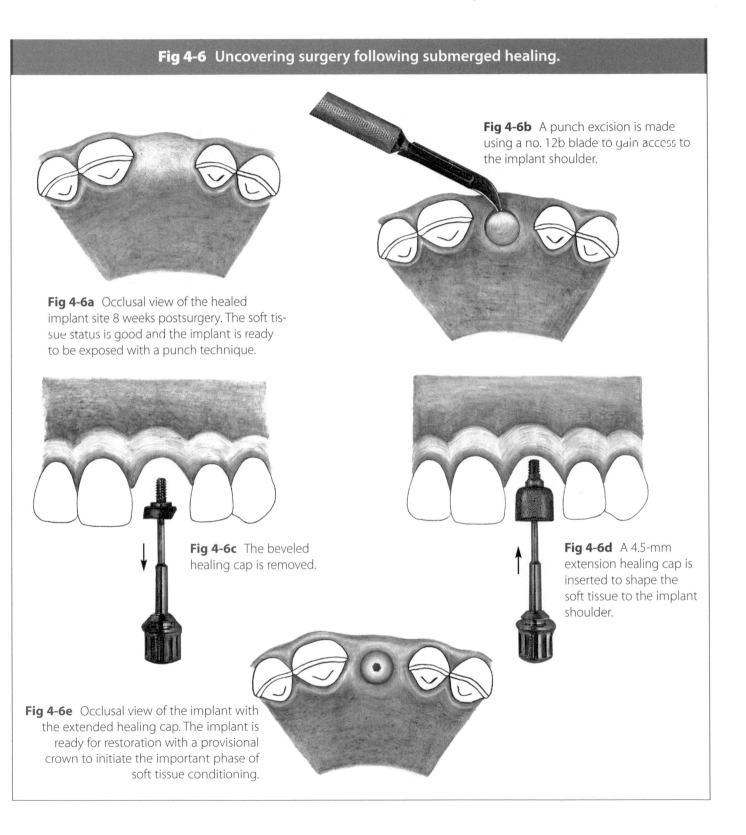

Fig 4-6 Uncovering surgery following submerged healing.

Fig 4-6b A punch excision is made using a no. 12b blade to gain access to the implant shoulder.

Fig 4-6a Occlusal view of the healed implant site 8 weeks postsurgery. The soft tissue status is good and the implant is ready to be exposed with a punch technique.

Fig 4-6c The beveled healing cap is removed.

Fig 4-6d A 4.5-mm extension healing cap is inserted to shape the soft tissue to the implant shoulder.

Fig 4-6e Occlusal view of the implant with the extended healing cap. The implant is ready for restoration with a provisional crown to initiate the important phase of soft tissue conditioning.

Fig 4-7 Flap elevation in a maxillary lateral incisor site.

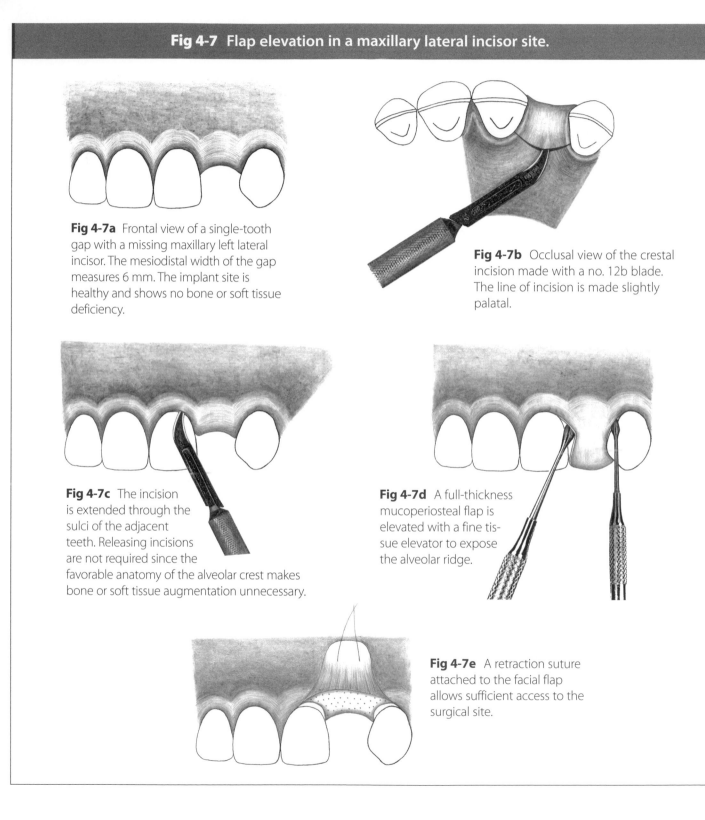

Fig 4-7a Frontal view of a single-tooth gap with a missing maxillary left lateral incisor. The mesiodistal width of the gap measures 6 mm. The implant site is healthy and shows no bone or soft tissue deficiency.

Fig 4-7b Occlusal view of the crestal incision made with a no. 12b blade. The line of incision is made slightly palatal.

Fig 4-7c The incision is extended through the sulci of the adjacent teeth. Releasing incisions are not required since the favorable anatomy of the alveolar crest makes bone or soft tissue augmentation unnecessary.

Fig 4-7d A full-thickness mucoperiosteal flap is elevated with a fine tissue elevator to expose the alveolar ridge.

Fig 4-7e A retraction suture attached to the facial flap allows sufficient access to the surgical site.

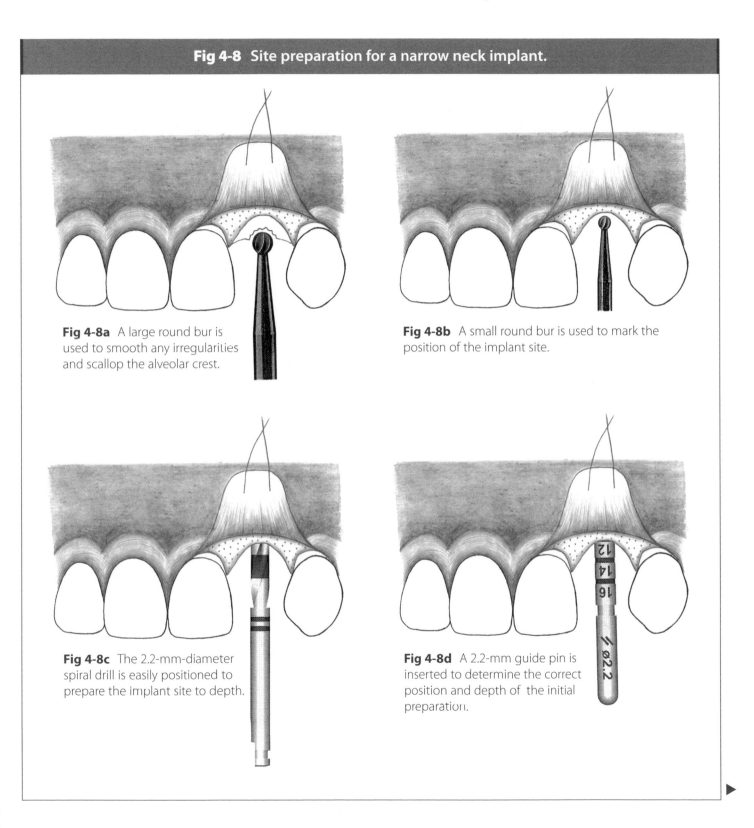

Fig 4-8 Site preparation for a narrow neck implant.

Fig 4-8a A large round bur is used to smooth any irregularities and scallop the alveolar crest.

Fig 4-8b A small round bur is used to mark the position of the implant site.

Fig 4-8c The 2.2-mm-diameter spiral drill is easily positioned to prepare the implant site to depth.

Fig 4-8d A 2.2-mm guide pin is inserted to determine the correct position and depth of the initial preparation.

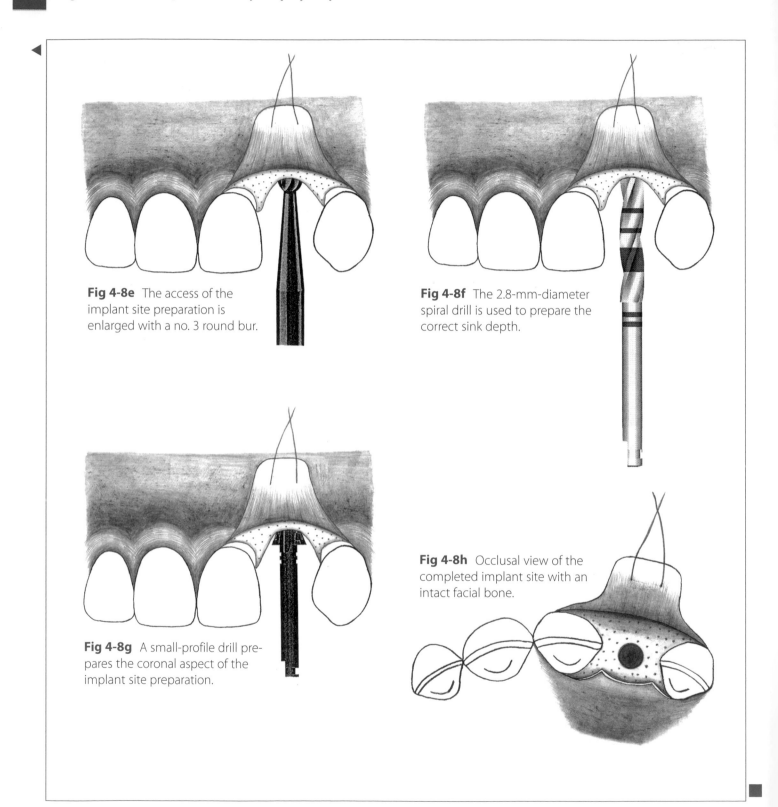

Fig 4-8e The access of the implant site preparation is enlarged with a no. 3 round bur.

Fig 4-8f The 2.8-mm-diameter spiral drill is used to prepare the correct sink depth.

Fig 4-8g A small-profile drill prepares the coronal aspect of the implant site preparation.

Fig 4-8h Occlusal view of the completed implant site with an intact facial bone.

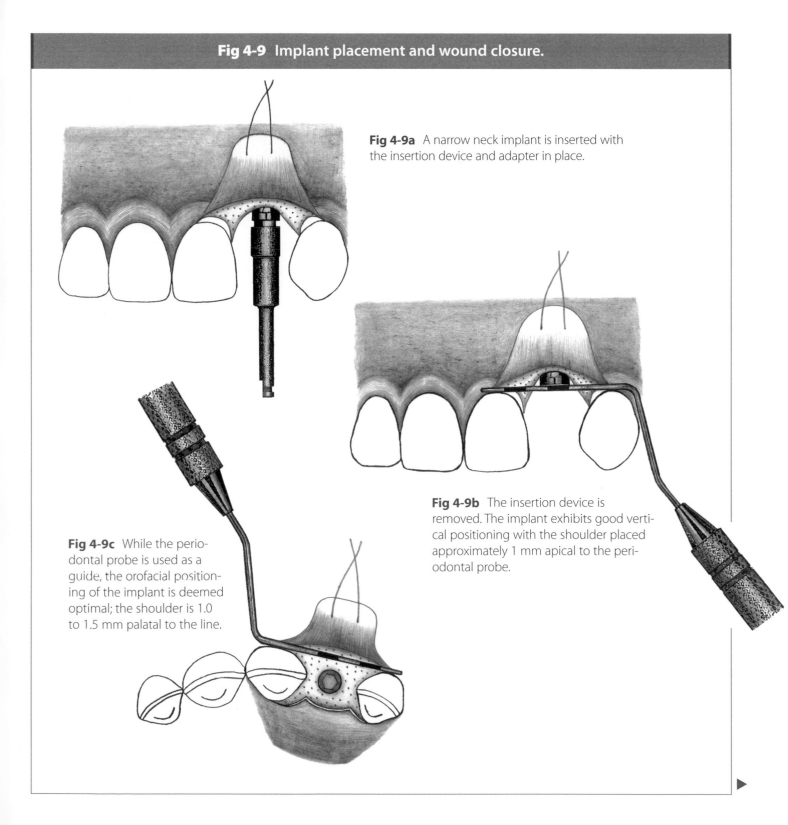

Fig 4-9 Implant placement and wound closure.

Fig 4-9a A narrow neck implant is inserted with the insertion device and adapter in place.

Fig 4-9b The insertion device is removed. The implant exhibits good vertical positioning with the shoulder placed approximately 1 mm apical to the periodontal probe.

Fig 4-9c While the periodontal probe is used as a guide, the orofacial positioning of the implant is deemed optimal; the shoulder is 1.0 to 1.5 mm palatal to the line.

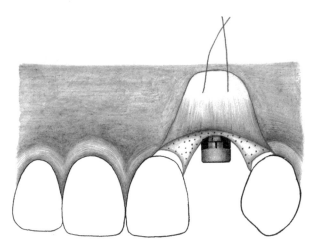

Fig 4-9d Final position of the narrow neck plus implant with a small healing cap in place.

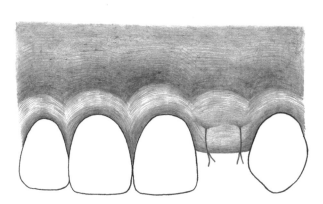

Fig 4-9e Closure of the surgical site using 5-0 interrupted single sutures.

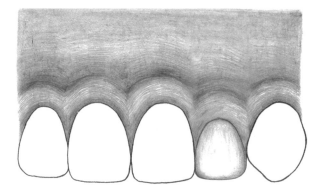

Fig 4-9f A provisional removable partial denture is adjusted and positioned over the missing maxillary lateral incisor site.

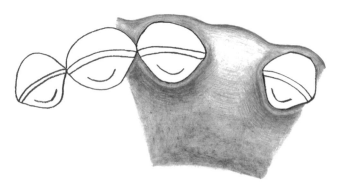

Fig 4-9g After 6 weeks, the surgical site demonstrates excellent soft tissue healing. The implant is ready to be exposed with a punch technique.

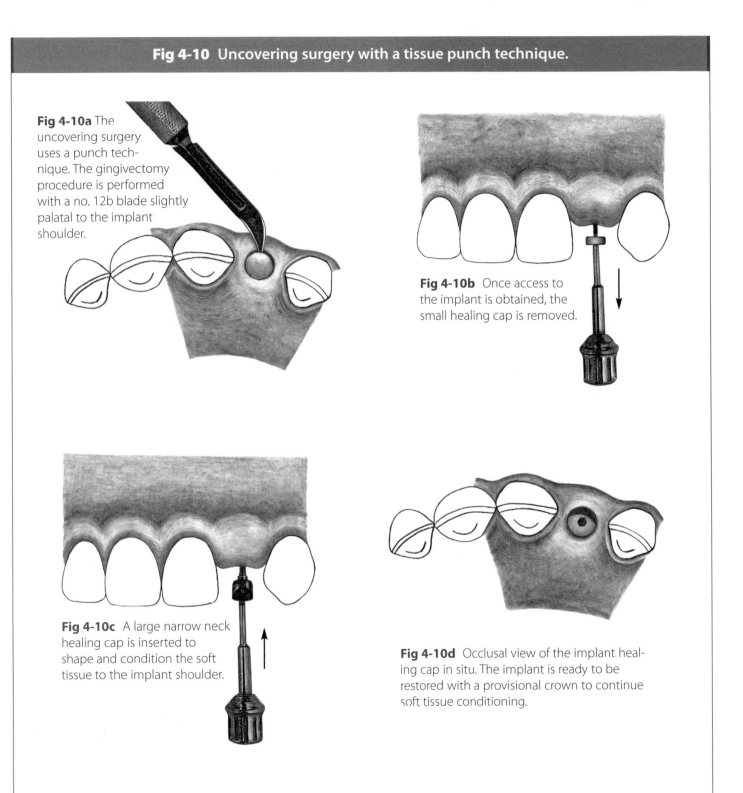

Fig 4-10 Uncovering surgery with a tissue punch technique.

Fig 4-10a The uncovering surgery uses a punch technique. The gingivectomy procedure is performed with a no. 12b blade slightly palatal to the implant shoulder.

Fig 4-10b Once access to the implant is obtained, the small healing cap is removed.

Fig 4-10c A large narrow neck healing cap is inserted to shape and condition the soft tissue to the implant shoulder.

Fig 4-10d Occlusal view of the implant healing cap in situ. The implant is ready to be restored with a provisional crown to continue soft tissue conditioning.

chapter 5

Surgical Procedures for Implant Placement with Simultaneous Guided Bone Regeneration

The presence of localized bone defects in the alveolar process of implant patients is a common clinical situation. Thus, surgical techniques have been developed to predictably augment bone deficiencies. One technique is based on the principle of guided bone regeneration (GBR) using barrier membranes. The so-called GBR technique has become a standard of care in daily practice. Today, bioabsorbable collagen membranes are preferred in GBR procedures because they offer several advantages, such as an easy clinical handling during surgery due to hydrophilic properties, a low risk for complications in case of a soft tissue dehiscence, and no need for a second surgical intervention for membrane removal. However, these soft membranes tend to collapse and have a rather short barrier function. To compensate for these disadvantages, collagen membranes are combined with appropriate bone fillers, such as a combination of autogenous bone chips and deproteinized bovine bone mineral (DBBM) that is applied in two layers.

This chapter presents the application of the current GBR technique in two typical clinical situations, an apical fenestration defect and a crestal dehiscence defect in an extraction socket using the concept of early implant placement.

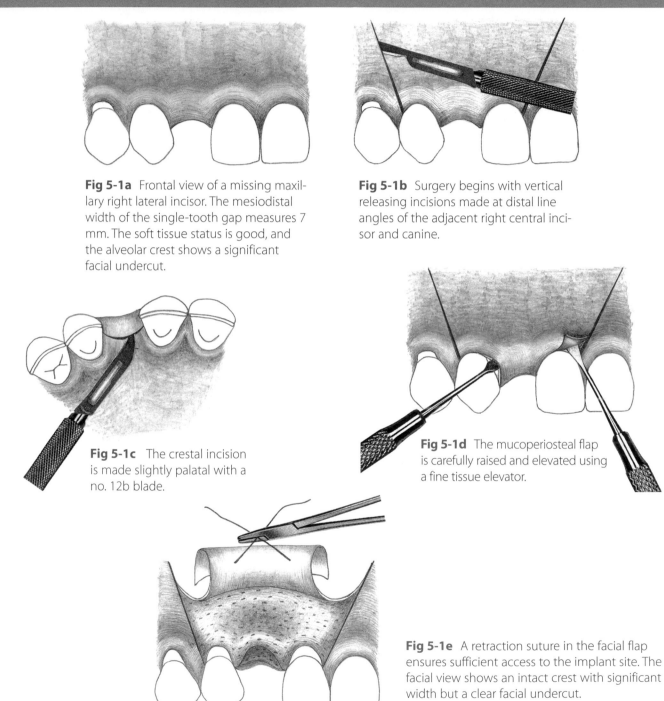

Fig 5-1 Flap elevation in an implant site with an apical fenestraton defect.

Fig 5-1a Frontal view of a missing maxillary right lateral incisor. The mesiodistal width of the single-tooth gap measures 7 mm. The soft tissue status is good, and the alveolar crest shows a significant facial undercut.

Fig 5-1b Surgery begins with vertical releasing incisions made at distal line angles of the adjacent right central incisor and canine.

Fig 5-1c The crestal incision is made slightly palatal with a no. 12b blade.

Fig 5-1d The mucoperiosteal flap is carefully raised and elevated using a fine tissue elevator.

Fig 5-1e A retraction suture in the facial flap ensures sufficient access to the implant site. The facial view shows an intact crest with significant width but a clear facial undercut.

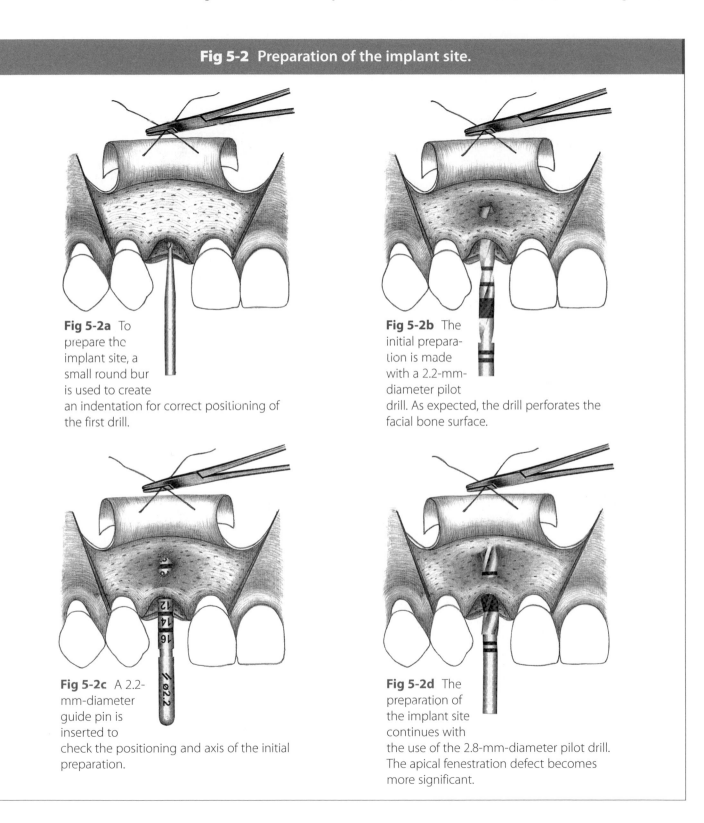

Fig 5-2 Preparation of the implant site.

Fig 5-2a To prepare the implant site, a small round bur is used to create an indentation for correct positioning of the first drill.

Fig 5-2b The initial preparation is made with a 2.2-mm-diameter pilot drill. As expected, the drill perforates the facial bone surface.

Fig 5-2c A 2.2-mm-diameter guide pin is inserted to check the positioning and axis of the initial preparation.

Fig 5-2d The preparation of the implant site continues with the use of the 2.8-mm-diameter pilot drill. The apical fenestration defect becomes more significant.

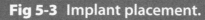

Fig 5-3 Implant placement.

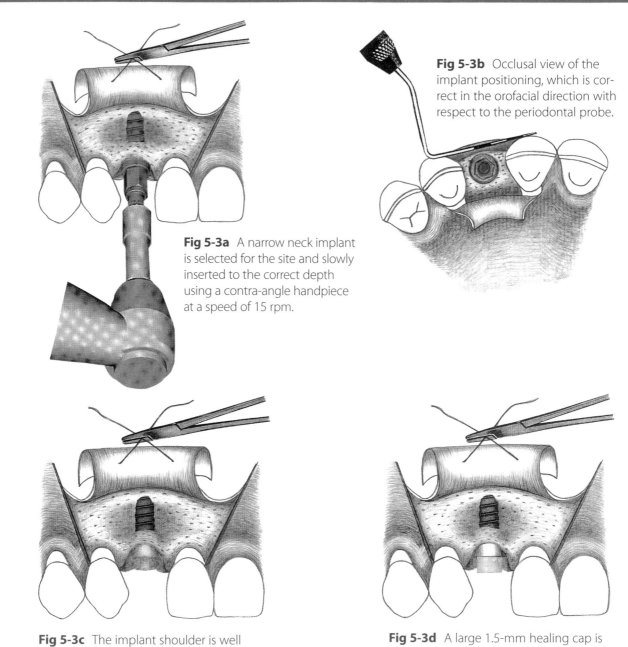

Fig 5-3a A narrow neck implant is selected for the site and slowly inserted to the correct depth using a contra-angle handpiece at a speed of 15 rpm.

Fig 5-3b Occlusal view of the implant positioning, which is correct in the orofacial direction with respect to the periodontal probe.

Fig 5-3c The implant shoulder is well positioned in the coronoapical direction, with the shoulder approximately 1 mm apical to the cementoenamel junction (CEJ) of adjacent teeth.

Fig 5-3d A large 1.5-mm healing cap is inserted to cover the shoulder of the narrow neck implant.

Fig 5-4 Simultaneous GBR in a site with an apical fenestration defect.

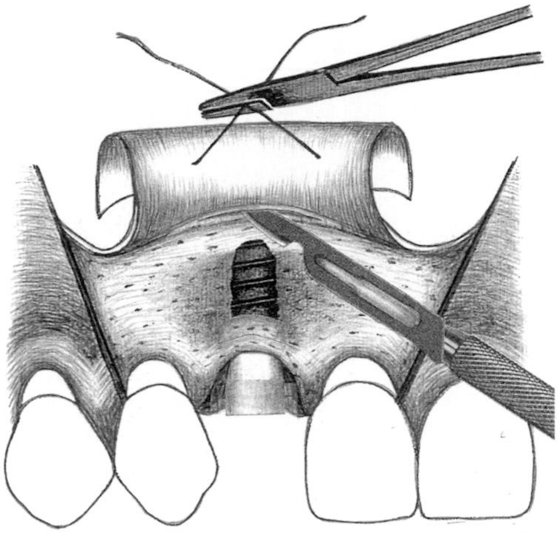

Fig 5-4a To ensure a tension-free primary wound closure, the periosteum is released with a new blade.

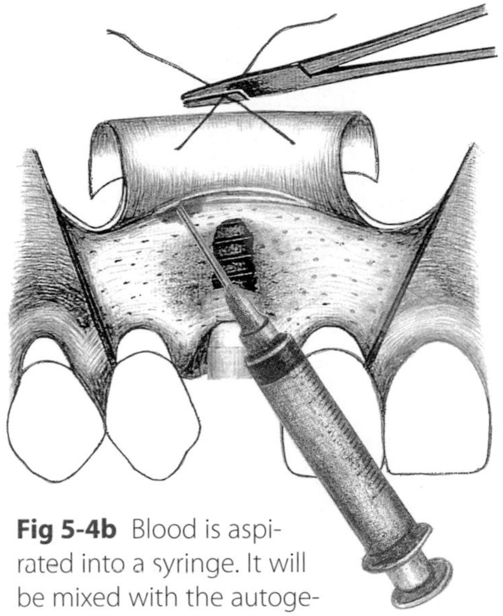

Fig 5-4b Blood is aspirated into a syringe. It will be mixed with the autogenous bone and DBBM granules for later use.

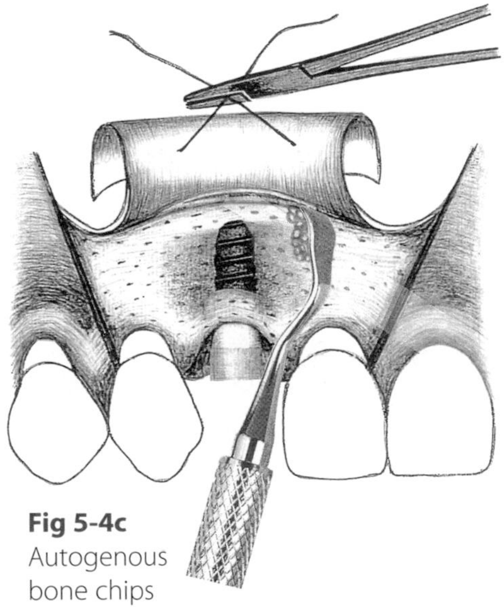

Fig 5-4c Autogenous bone chips are harvested from periapical bone surface using a bone scraper.

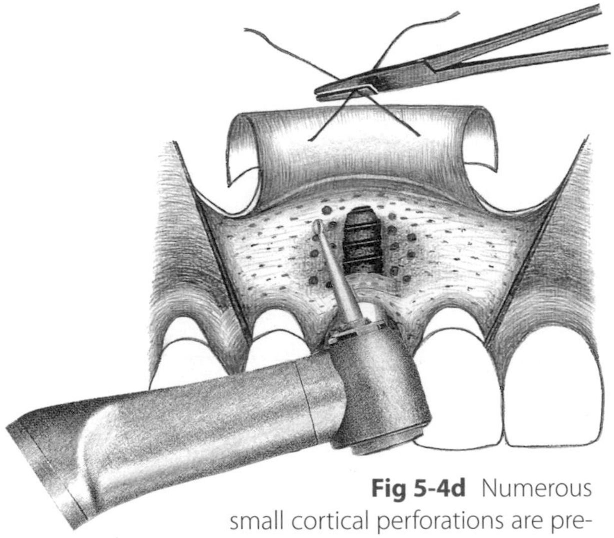

Fig 5-4d Numerous small cortical perforations are prepared around the apical fenestration defect to open the bone marrow cavity and facilitate the ingrowth of blood vessels during initial stages of bone healing.

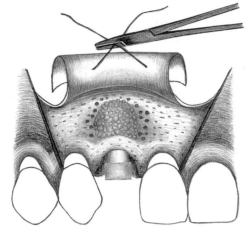

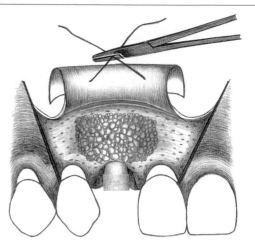

Fig 5-4e The autogenous bone chips are placed into the defect site to cover the exposed implant surface.

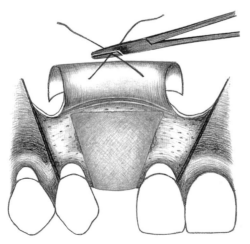

Fig 5-4g A resorbable collagen membrane is trimmed to the required shape using a pair of scissors. The membrane is cut into two strips, a smaller strip and a larger strip.

Fig 5-4f DBBM granules soaked in blood are placed over the autografts to rebuild the facial bone wall for soft tissue support. DBBM granules better maintain the volume of the alveolar process due to the low substitution rate of the bone filler.

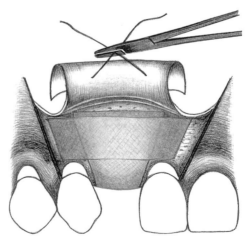

Fig 5-4h The larger membrane is placed over the graft and adapted to the site. Once it is soaked in blood, the membrane becomes self adhesive and stabilizes itself.

Fig 5-4i The smaller strip of membrane is trimmed for placement over the first membrane. This double-layer technique improves the stability of both membranes.

Fig 5-5 Wound closure for submerged healing.

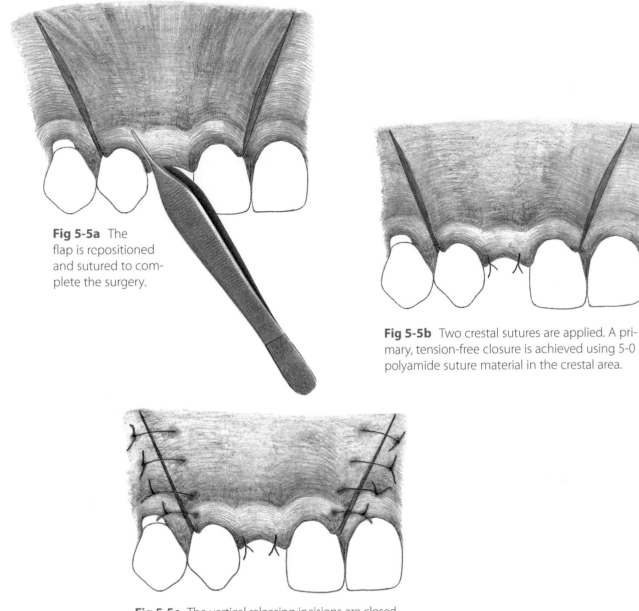

Fig 5-5a The flap is repositioned and sutured to complete the surgery.

Fig 5-5b Two crestal sutures are applied. A primary, tension-free closure is achieved using 5-0 polyamide suture material in the crestal area.

Fig 5-5c The vertical releasing incisions are closed with several interrupted single sutures using 6-0 suture material. After 8 weeks of healing, an implant uncovering procedure is performed as shown in Fig 4-10.

Fig 5-6 **Low-trauma tooth extraction without flap elevation.**

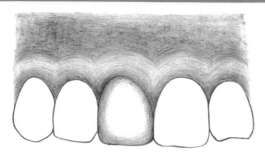

Fig 5-6a Frontal view of an unsalvageable maxillary right central incisor.

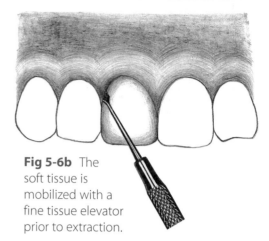

Fig 5-6b The soft tissue is mobilized with a fine tissue elevator prior to extraction.

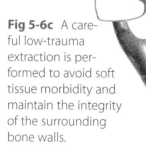

Fig 5-6c A careful low-trauma extraction is performed to avoid soft tissue morbidity and maintain the integrity of the surrounding bone walls.

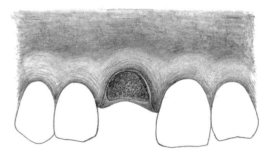

Fig 5-6d A collagen sponge is placed in the extraction socket to improve hemostasis.

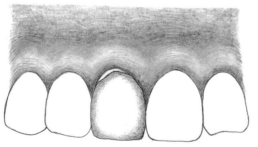

Fig 5-6e A provisional removable partial denture is trimmed and adjusted using an acrylic bur to prevent excessive pressure on the extraction site during the healing phase.

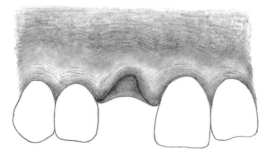

Fig 5-6f Eight weeks following extraction, the soft tissues are healed, and the facial bone wall shows a minor concavity.

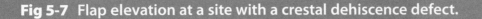

Fig 5-7 Flap elevation at a site with a crestal dehiscence defect.

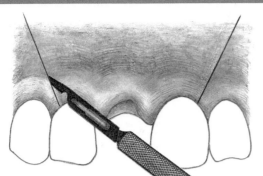

Fig 5-7a Surgery begins with vertical releasing incisions made at distal line angles of the adjacent right lateral incisor and left central incisor.

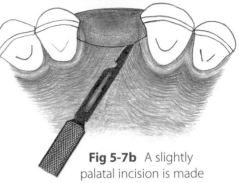

Fig 5-7b A slightly palatal incision is made in the crestal region using a no. 15c blade.

Fig 5-7c The mucoperiosteal flap is carefully raised and elevated using a fine tissue elevator.

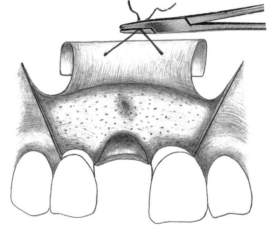

Fig 5-7d A retraction suture in the facial flap ensures sufficient access to the implant site. The facial view of the implant site exhibits a partially filled alveolus and a slight craterlike defect with respect to the levels of the CEJ of adjacent teeth.

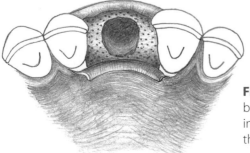

Fig 5-7e The occlusal view demonstrates a thin facial bone wall but no flattening of the alveolar ridge. Correct implant placement will result in a small two-wall defect on the facial aspect.

Fig 5-8 Preparation of the implant site.

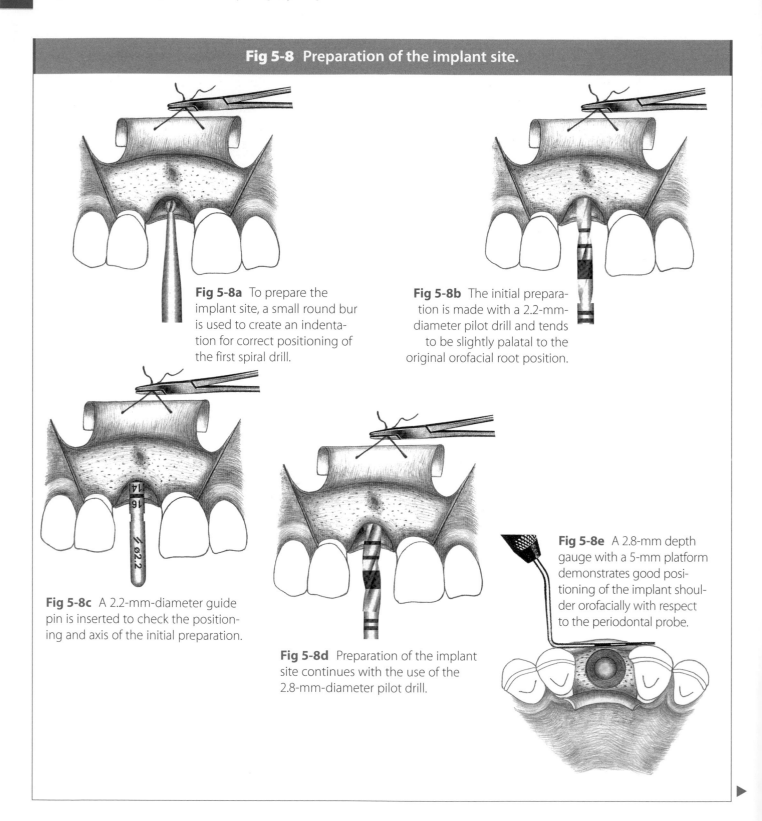

Fig 5-8a To prepare the implant site, a small round bur is used to create an indentation for correct positioning of the first spiral drill.

Fig 5-8b The initial preparation is made with a 2.2-mm-diameter pilot drill and tends to be slightly palatal to the original orofacial root position.

Fig 5-8c A 2.2-mm-diameter guide pin is inserted to check the positioning and axis of the initial preparation.

Fig 5-8d Preparation of the implant site continues with the use of the 2.8-mm-diameter pilot drill.

Fig 5-8e A 2.8-mm depth gauge with a 5-mm platform demonstrates good positioning of the implant shoulder orofacially with respect to the periodontal probe.

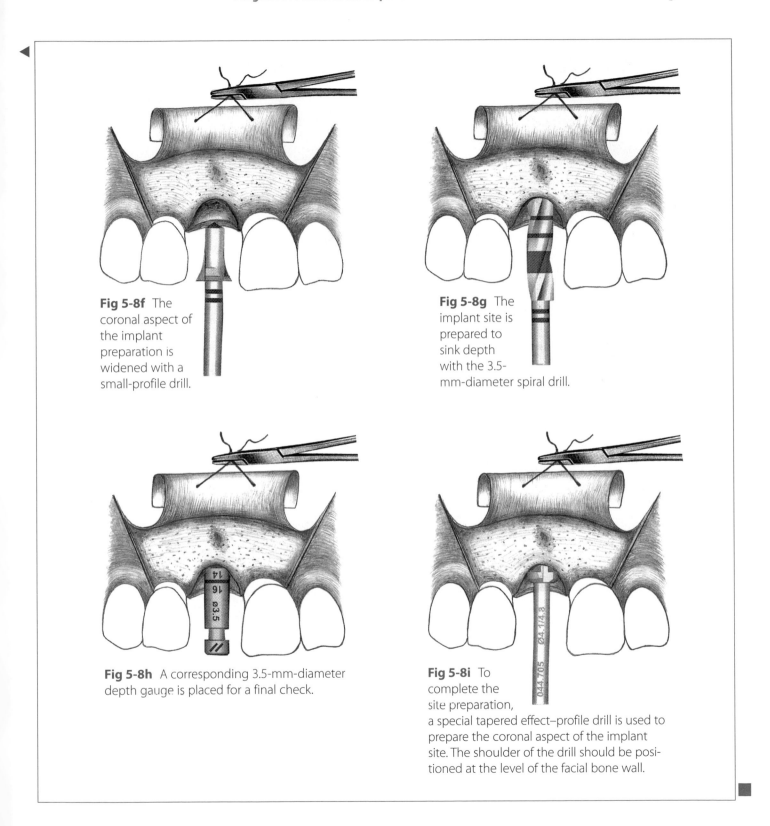

Fig 5-8f The coronal aspect of the implant preparation is widened with a small-profile drill.

Fig 5-8g The implant site is prepared to sink depth with the 3.5-mm-diameter spiral drill.

Fig 5-8h A corresponding 3.5-mm-diameter depth gauge is placed for a final check.

Fig 5-8i To complete the site preparation, a special tapered effect–profile drill is used to prepare the coronal aspect of the implant site. The shoulder of the drill should be positioned at the level of the facial bone wall.

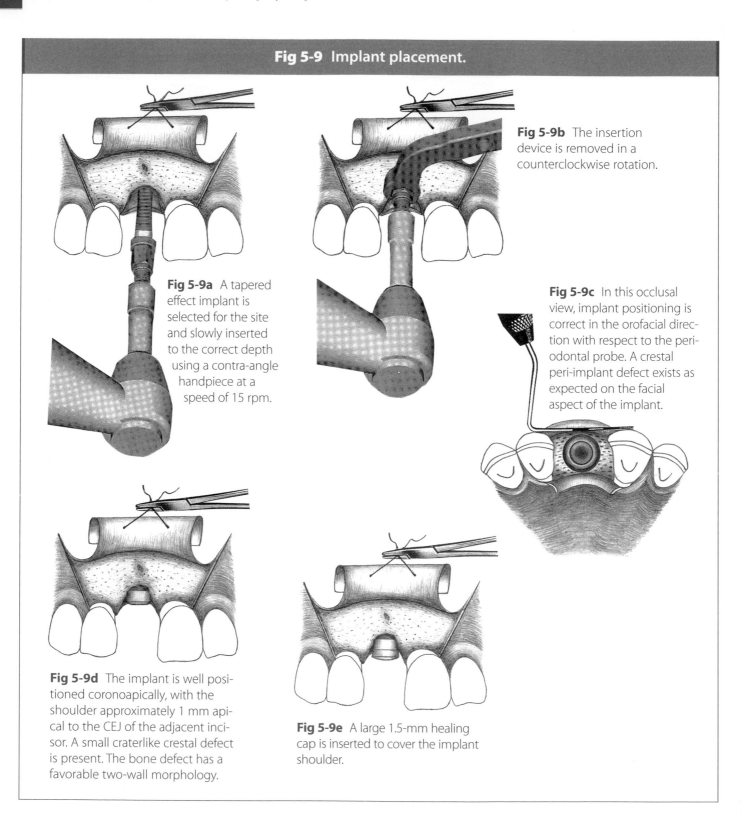

Fig 5-9 Implant placement.

Fig 5-9a A tapered effect implant is selected for the site and slowly inserted to the correct depth using a contra-angle handpiece at a speed of 15 rpm.

Fig 5-9b The insertion device is removed in a counterclockwise rotation.

Fig 5-9c In this occlusal view, implant positioning is correct in the orofacial direction with respect to the periodontal probe. A crestal peri-implant defect exists as expected on the facial aspect of the implant.

Fig 5-9d The implant is well positioned coronoapically, with the shoulder approximately 1 mm apical to the CEJ of the adjacent incisor. A small craterlike crestal defect is present. The bone defect has a favorable two-wall morphology.

Fig 5-9e A large 1.5-mm healing cap is inserted to cover the implant shoulder.

Fig 5-10 Simultaneous GBR in a site with a crestal dehiscence defect.

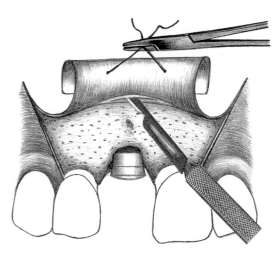

Fig 5-10a The periosteum is released with a new blade to ensure a tension-free primary wound closure.

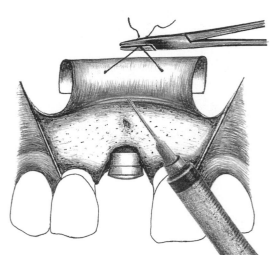

Fig 5-10b Blood is aspirated into a syringe. It will be mixed with the autogenous bone and DBBM granules for later use.

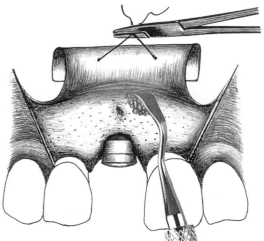

Fig 5-10c Autogenous bone chips are harvested from the nasal spine using a bone scraper.

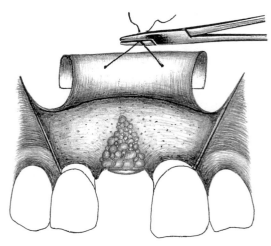

Fig 5-10d The autogenous bone chips are used to fill the peri-implant bone defect and cover the exposed implant surface.

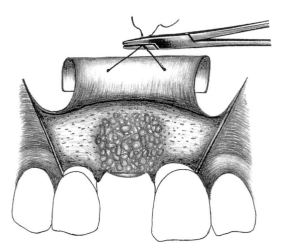

Fig 5-10e The DBBM-blood mixture is placed over the autografts and the alveolar process. The goal is to build up the facial bone wall to support the soft tissues, creating a convex contour.

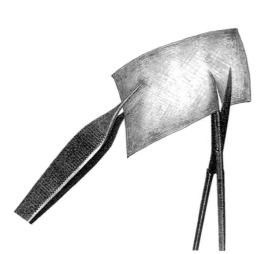

Fig 5-10f A resorbable collagen membrane is trimmed to the required shape using a pair of scissors. The membrane is cut into two strips, a smaller strip and a larger strip.

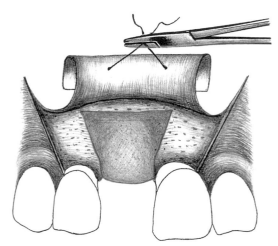

Fig 5-10g The larger membrane is placed over the grafted site and adapted to the surrounding bone. Once it is soaked in blood, the membrane becomes self adhesive and stabilizes itself.

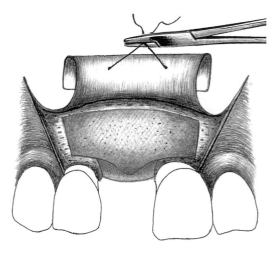

Fig 5-10h The smaller strip of membrane is positioned over the first membrane. This double-layer technique improves the stability of both membranes.

Fig 5-11 Wound closure for submerged healing.

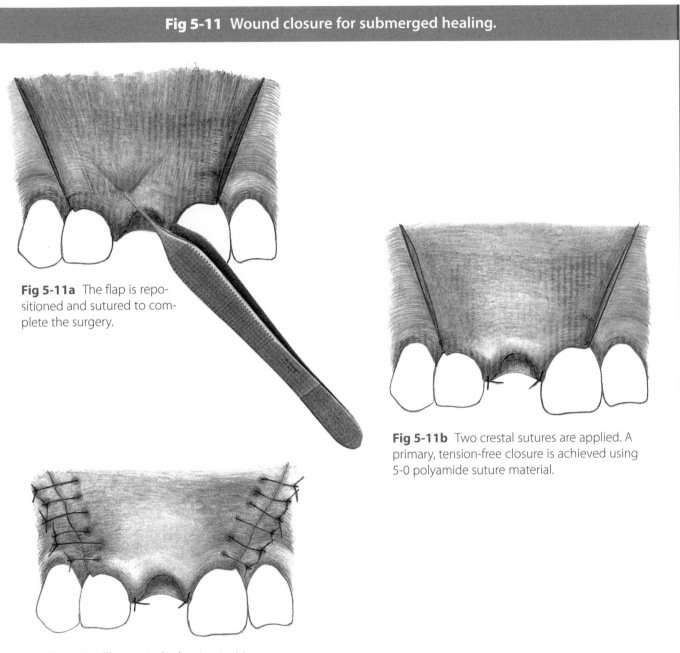

Fig 5-11a The flap is repositioned and sutured to complete the surgery.

Fig 5-11b Two crestal sutures are applied. A primary, tension-free closure is achieved using 5-0 polyamide suture material.

Fig 5-11c The vertical releasing incisions on the facial aspects are closed with several interrupted single sutures. After 8 weeks of healing, the patient is scheduled for the implant uncovering procedure prior to prosthetic restoration.

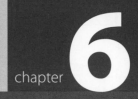
Surgical Procedures for Implant Placement with Simultaneous Sinus Floor Elevation

Insufficient alveolar bone height for implant placement is an oft-seen problem in the posterior maxilla. Two surgical techniques for sinus floor elevation are frequently used to overcome this local bone deficiency: the lateral window technique and the osteotome technique.

Sinus floor elevation via the lateral window technique, developed in the 1970s, is predominantly used either with a simultaneous or staged approach for implant placement. Whenever possible, a simultaneous implant placement is recommended to eliminate a second surgical procedure for the patient. The most important prerequisite is an alveolar bone height of at least 5 mm to allow implant placement with good primary stability. When alveolar bone height is less than 5 mm, a staged approach is necessary. Following preparation of the facial bony window and careful mobilization of the sinus membrane, a mixture of autogenous bone graft and a bone substitute with a low substitution rate is applied to elevate the mucous membrane apically. The lateral window technique easily allows a gain in alveolar bone height between 8 and 15 mm.

The sinus floor elevation via the osteotome technique, developed in the 1990s, is an alternative to the lateral window technique but can only be used if the local anatomy meets certain prerequisites. The technique requires an initial alveolar bone height of at least 5 mm and a flat anatomy of the sinus floor in both the mesiodistal and orofacial directions. The local anatomy must be examined with a three-dimensional radiographic technique, such as a digital volume (cone-beam) tomography or a dental computed tomography scan. In addition, the gain in alveolar bone height is limited to 4 to 7 mm.

The chapter presents two typical indications for sinus floor elevation in the posterior maxilla: a distal extension situation and a single-tooth replacement in a first molar site.

Fig 6-1 Preoperative evaluation for the lateral window technique.

Fig 6-1a Facial view of a long-span distal extension situation in the right maxilla.

Fig 6-1b Radiographic view showing the preoperative situation with insufficient bone height in the posterior maxilla. The treatment plan involves placing two implants in the premolar sites to allow simultaneous sinus floor elevation using the window technique.

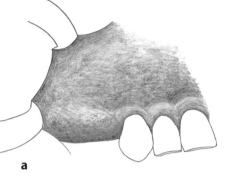

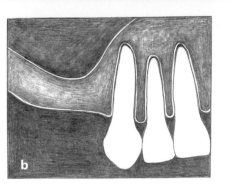

Fig 6-2 Flap elevation in the posterior maxilla.

Fig 6-2a Following a midcrestal incision, intrasulcular and vertical releasing incisions are made mesial to the line angle of the maxillary right canine.

Fig 6-2b With a fine tissue elevator, the entire flap is carefully elevated to expose the surgical site beneath.

Fig 6-2c Retraction sutures are placed on the facial and palatal flaps.

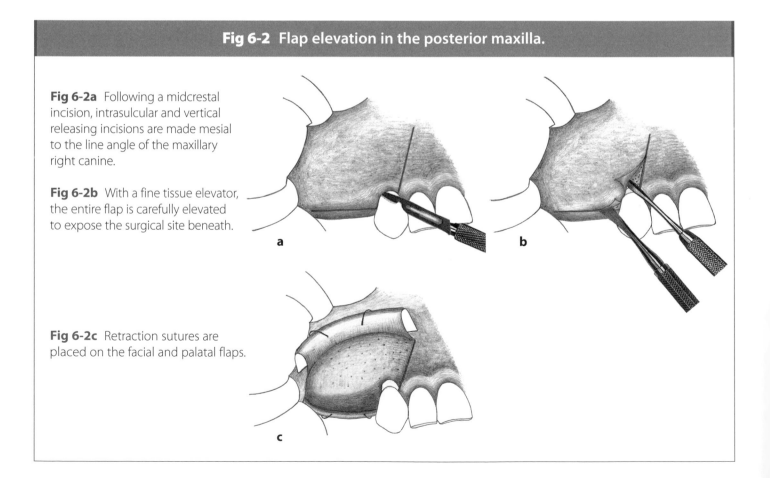

Fig 6-3 Preparation of the lateral bone window.

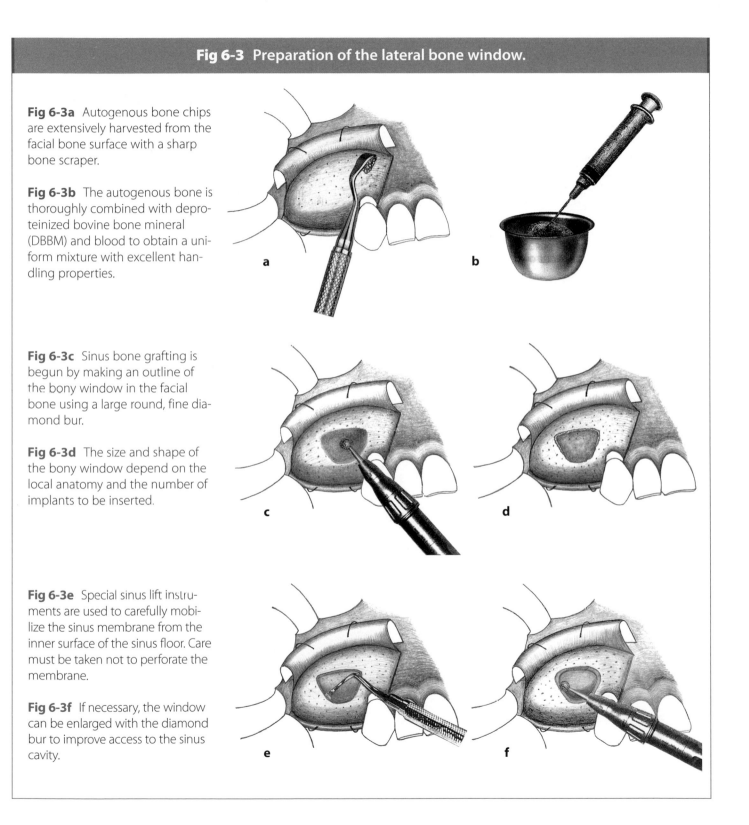

Fig 6-3a Autogenous bone chips are extensively harvested from the facial bone surface with a sharp bone scraper.

Fig 6-3b The autogenous bone is thoroughly combined with deproteinized bovine bone mineral (DBBM) and blood to obtain a uniform mixture with excellent handling properties.

Fig 6-3c Sinus bone grafting is begun by making an outline of the bony window in the facial bone using a large round, fine diamond bur.

Fig 6-3d The size and shape of the bony window depend on the local anatomy and the number of implants to be inserted.

Fig 6-3e Special sinus lift instruments are used to carefully mobilize the sinus membrane from the inner surface of the sinus floor. Care must be taken not to perforate the membrane.

Fig 6-3f If necessary, the window can be enlarged with the diamond bur to improve access to the sinus cavity.

Fig 6-4 Site preparation for implant placement.

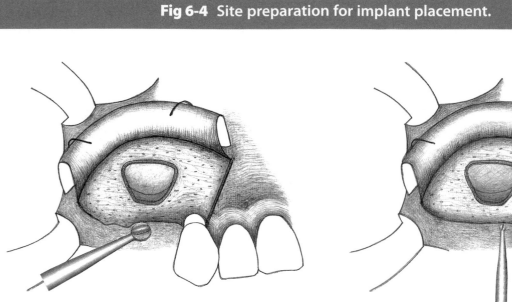

Fig 6-4a Preparation of the implant sites begins with smoothing the crest of the alveolar ridge with a large round bur.

Fig 6-4b Indentations of the implant surgical sites are created with a small round bur.

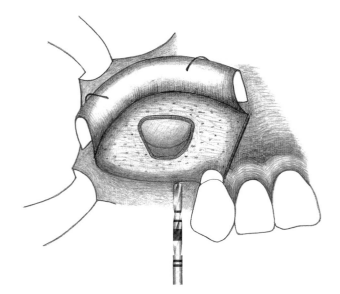
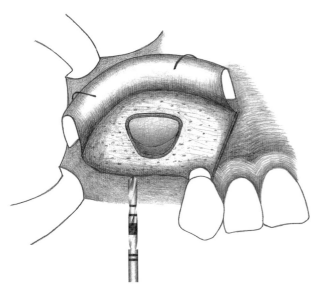

Fig 6-4c The implant sites are prepared using a 2.2-mm-diameter pilot drill, beginning with the most anterior implant site.

Fig 6-4d The second implant site is subsequently prepared.

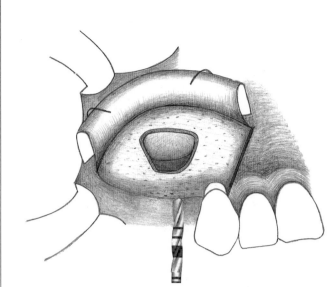

Fig 6-4e A 2.8-mm-diameter spiral drill is easily inserted and prepared to depth.

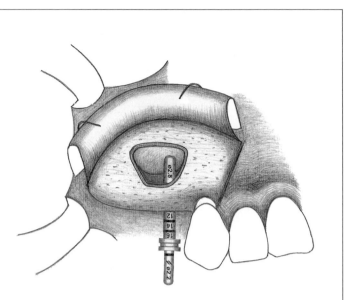

Fig 6-4f The 2.8-mm-diameter depth gauge is inserted and the implant site positioning and axis are checked.

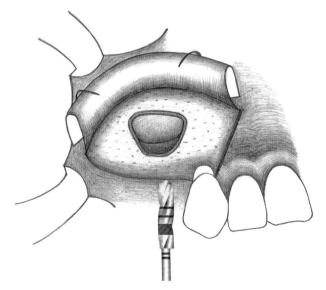

Fig 6-4g The site is prepared with the 3.5-mm-diameter spiral drill.

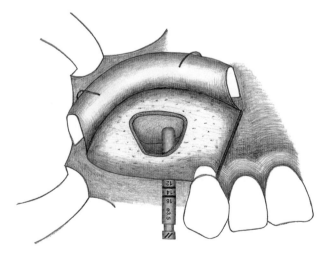

Fig 6-4h The implant bed and its position are checked with the corresponding 3.5-mm-diameter depth gauge.

Fig 6-5 Sinus bone grafting and simultaneous implant placement.

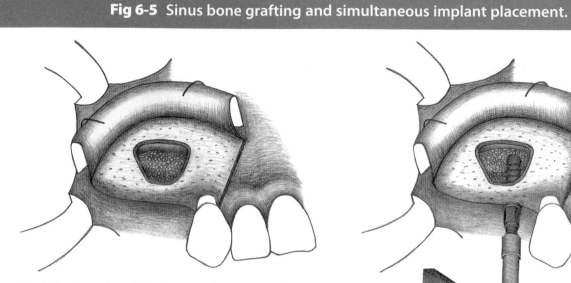

Fig 6-5a A portion of the bone-graft mixture is placed into the interior-most part of the bony window against the newly elevated sinus membrane. It is also applied in the regions of the future implant positions.

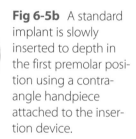

Fig 6-5b A standard implant is slowly inserted to depth in the first premolar position using a contra-angle handpiece attached to the insertion device.

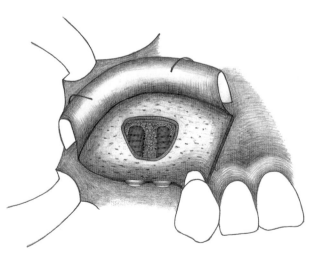

Fig 6-5c A wide body implant is inserted in the second premolar position. It is important to achieve primary stability to ensure osseointegration of both implants during the initial healing period.

Fig 6-5d Once the implants are inserted to depth, the insertion devices are removed and closure screws are placed.

Fig 6-5e The remaining bone–graft mixture is packed to fill the bony window and cover the exposed implant surfaces.

Fig 6-5f A resorbable collagen membrane is trimmed to the required shape using a pair of scissors.

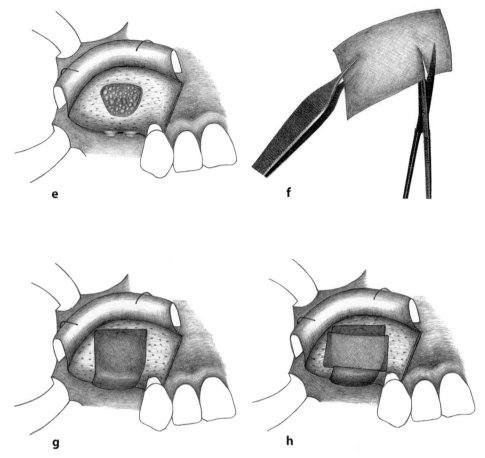

e

f

Fig 6-5g The membrane is placed over the grafted bony window and adapted to the surgical site. Once it is soaked in blood, the membrane becomes self adhesive and stabilizes itself.

Fig 6-5h A second strip of membrane is cut and positioned on top of the first one. This double-layer technique improves the stability of both membranes.

g

h

Fig 6-5i Following flap repositioning, flap closure is achieved with numerous interrupted single sutures.

Fig 6-5j Postoperative radiographic view showing the two implants and bone augmentation material applied to gain additional height in the alveolar bone. A healing period of 12 weeks is recommended before implant restoration.

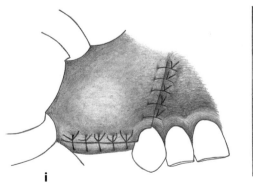

i

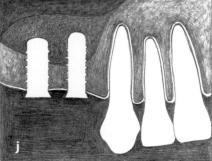

j

Fig 6-6 Preoperative evaluation for the osteotome technique.

Fig 6-6a Occlusal view of a single-tooth gap in the maxilla due to a missing first molar. The alveolar crest width is sufficient for the placement of a wide neck implant.

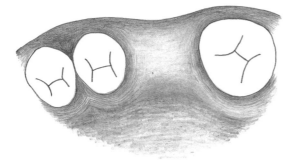

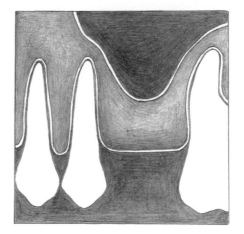

Fig 6-6b Anatomic prerequisites for the osteotome technique. The schematic diagram shows an alveolar bone height of approximately 7 mm and a flat sinus floor in the mesiodistal direction.

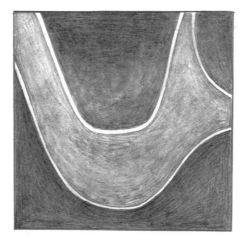

Fig 6-6c The radiographic cross section confirms a flat sinus floor anatomy in the lateral direction.

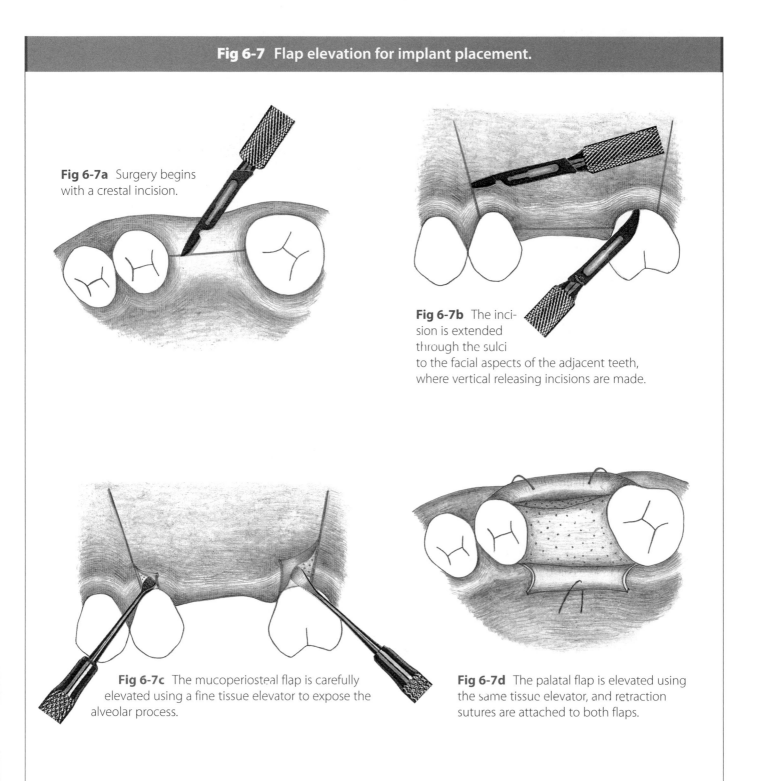

Fig 6-7 Flap elevation for implant placement.

Fig 6-7a Surgery begins with a crestal incision.

Fig 6-7b The incision is extended through the sulci to the facial aspects of the adjacent teeth, where vertical releasing incisions are made.

Fig 6-7c The mucoperiosteal flap is carefully elevated using a fine tissue elevator to expose the alveolar process.

Fig 6-7d The palatal flap is elevated using the same tissue elevator, and retraction sutures are attached to both flaps.

Fig 6-8 Site preparation for implant placement.

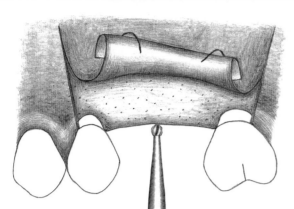

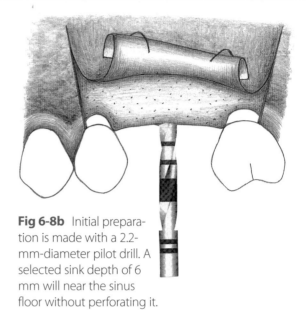

Fig 6-8a A small round bur is used to create an indentation for correct positioning of the first pilot drill.

Fig 6-8b Initial preparation is made with a 2.2-mm-diameter pilot drill. A selected sink depth of 6 mm will near the sinus floor without perforating it.

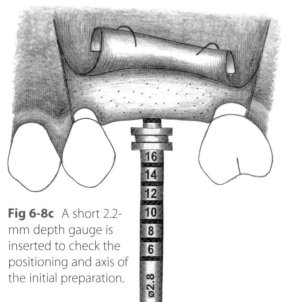

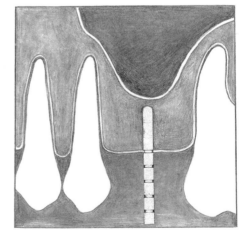

Fig 6-8c A short 2.2-mm depth gauge is inserted to check the positioning and axis of the initial preparation.

Fig 6-8d A periapical radiograph is taken to assess the distance of the preparation to the roots of the adjacent teeth and, more importantly, to the sinus floor. The radiograph reveals good angulation of the depth gauge and a 1-mm distance to the sinus floor.

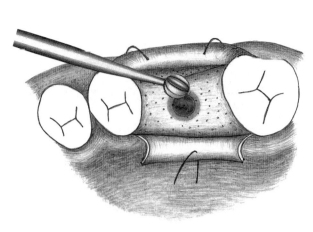

Fig 6-8e A large round bur is used to widen the surgical access.

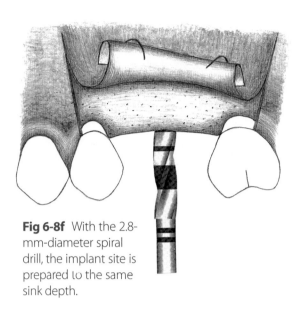

Fig 6-8f With the 2.8-mm-diameter spiral drill, the implant site is prepared to the same sink depth.

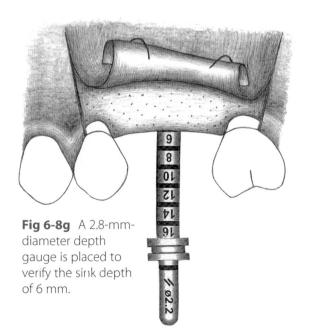

Fig 6-8g A 2.8-mm-diameter depth gauge is placed to verify the sink depth of 6 mm.

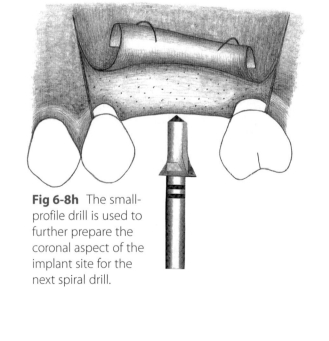

Fig 6-8h The small-profile drill is used to further prepare the coronal aspect of the implant site for the next spiral drill.

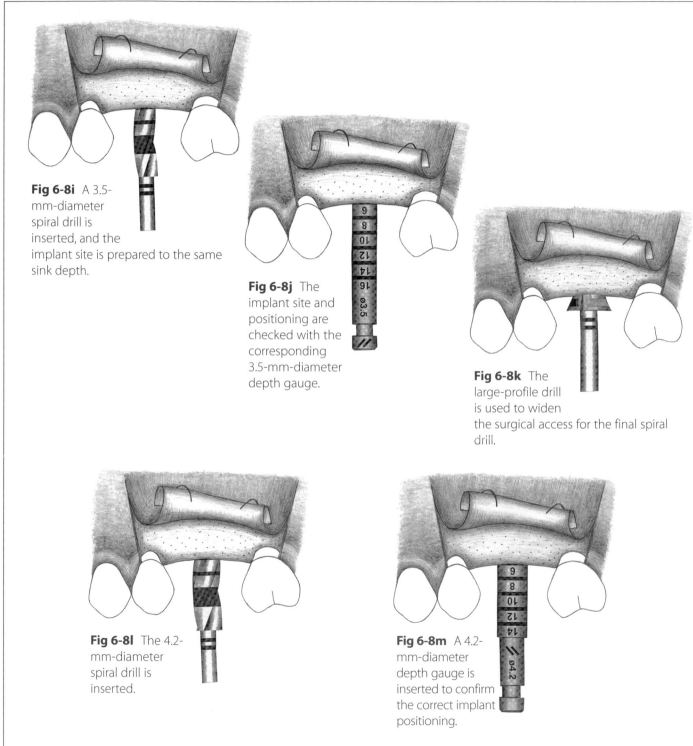

Fig 6-8i A 3.5-mm-diameter spiral drill is inserted, and the implant site is prepared to the same sink depth.

Fig 6-8j The implant site and positioning are checked with the corresponding 3.5-mm-diameter depth gauge.

Fig 6-8k The large-profile drill is used to widen the surgical access for the final spiral drill.

Fig 6-8l The 4.2-mm-diameter spiral drill is inserted.

Fig 6-8m A 4.2-mm-diameter depth gauge is inserted to confirm the correct implant positioning.

Fig 6-9 Osteotome technique in preparation for implant placement.

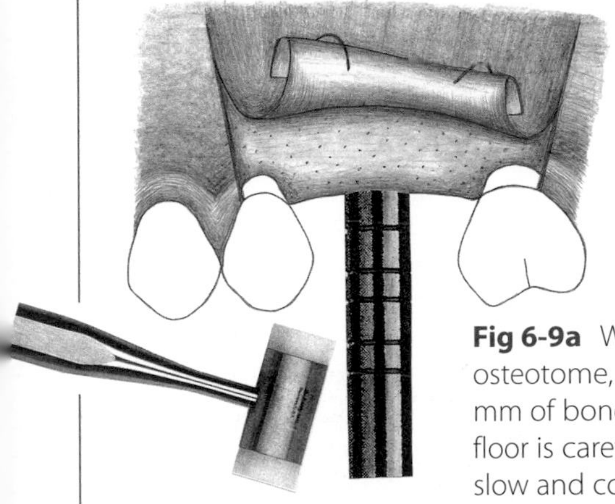

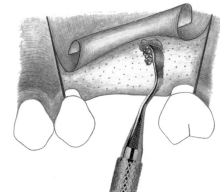

Fig 6-9a With a mallet and an osteotome, the remaining 1 mm of bone apical to the sinus floor is carefully infractured in a slow and controlled motion. A change in tapping sound from light to dull indicates the fracture of the thin sinus floor.

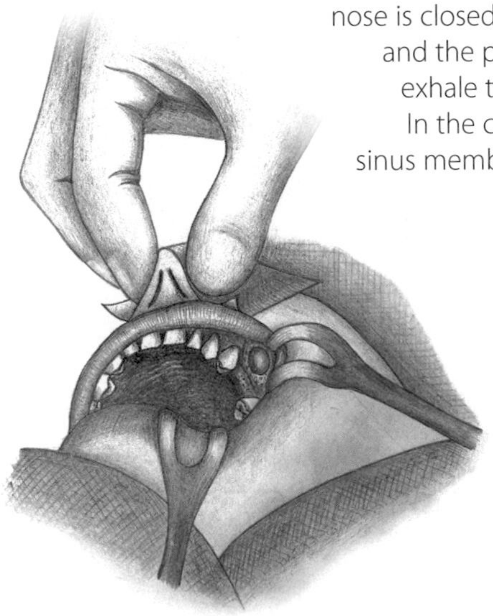

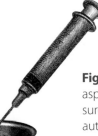

Fig 6-9b The intact sinus membrane is checked with the nose blow test. The nose is closed with two fingers and the patient is asked to exhale through the nose. In the case of a ruptured sinus membrane, a noise will be apparent.

Fig 6-9c Autogenous bone chips are harvested from the facial bone surface with a bone scraper and placed in a sterile dish.

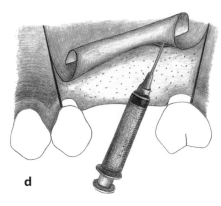

d

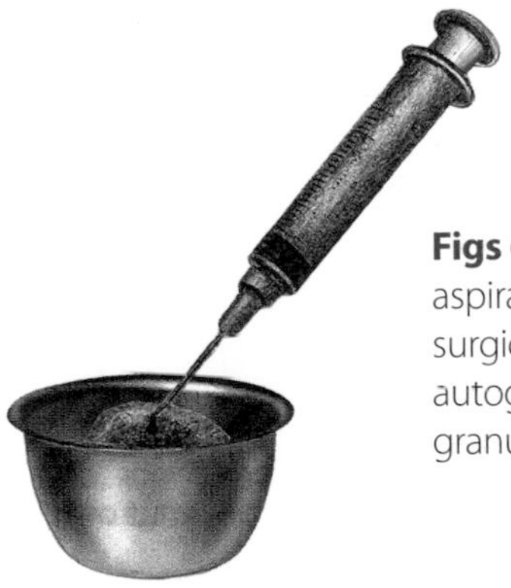

e

Figs 6-9d and 6-9e Blood is aspirated from the surrounding surgical site and mixed with the autogenous bone graft and DBBM granules in a ratio of 1:1.

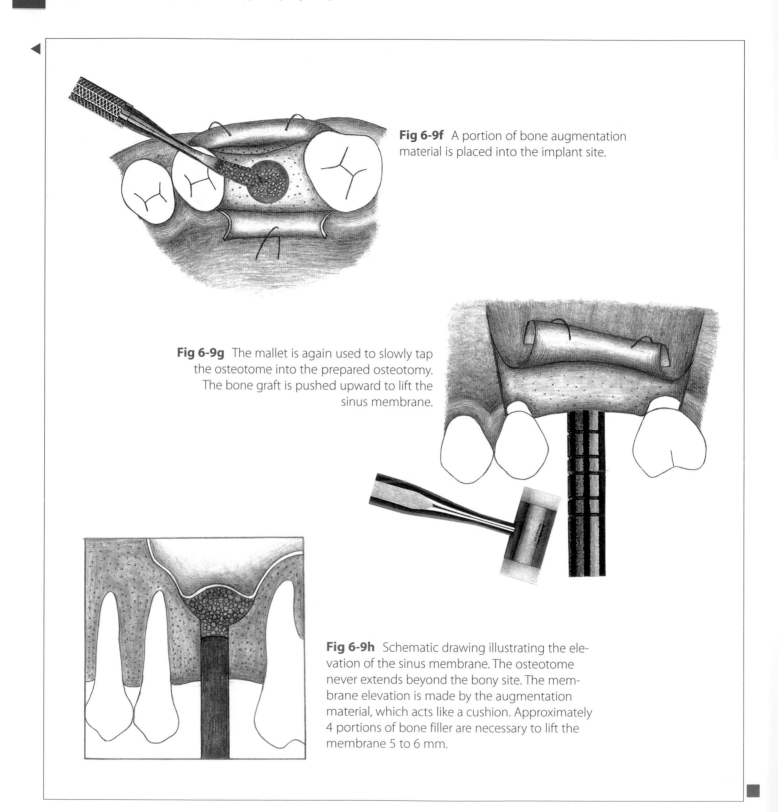

Fig 6-9f A portion of bone augmentation material is placed into the implant site.

Fig 6-9g The mallet is again used to slowly tap the osteotome into the prepared osteotomy. The bone graft is pushed upward to lift the sinus membrane.

Fig 6-9h Schematic drawing illustrating the elevation of the sinus membrane. The osteotome never extends beyond the bony site. The membrane elevation is made by the augmentation material, which acts like a cushion. Approximately 4 portions of bone filler are necessary to lift the membrane 5 to 6 mm.

Fig 6-10 Implant placement following sinus floor elevation.

Fig 6-10a A 10-mm wide neck implant is slowly inserted to the correct depth using a contra-angle handpiece at a speed of 15 rpm.

Fig 6-10b The insertion device is removed in a counterclockwise rotation.

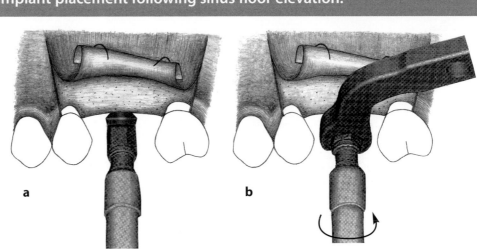

a

b

Fig 6-10c A 3-mm healing cap is attached to the implant to extend the implant above the soft tissue level and allow for a nonsubmerged healing.

Fig 6-10d To complete the surgery, the flap is repositioned and sutured crestally with two interrupted single sutures.

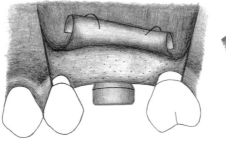

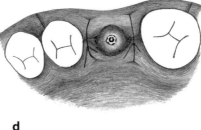

c

d

Fig 6-10e Finally, several interrupted single sutures close the releasing incisions.

Fig 6-10f Schematic cross section showing the 10-mm wide neck implant in place and the elevated sinus membrane following the application of bone augmentation material. The healing period will take 8 weeks before the implant can be restored with a single crown.

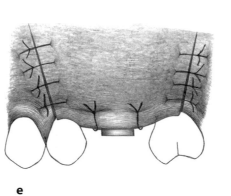

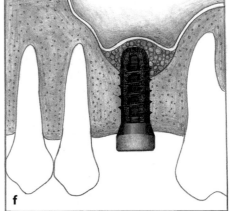

e

f

chapter 7

Clinical Cases

This chapter presents 14 clinical cases treated by the authors using the step-by-step surgical techniques described and illustrated in the preceding 6 chapters. Standard implant placement without bone grafting is demonstrated in the first 9 patients; the other 5 patients had local bone deficiencies that required bone augmentation performed at the same time as implant placement. In addition to the procedures themselves, the clinical photographs presented in these cases document long-term follow-ups extending for a period of up to 10 years in most standard implant cases, offering compelling evidence of the successful long-term outcome of the procedures when applied in daily practice. Developed in the late 1990s, the simultaneous bone augmentation procedures today represent an integral component of the authors' daily practice routine.

The authors would like to acknowledge their colleagues for the restorative work featured in the clinical cases: Dr Christian Balsiger, Wattenwil, Switzerland (case 1); Dr Dieter Müller, Bremgarten, Switzerland (case 2); Dr Claudio Schmid, Bern, Switzerland (case 4); Dr Bruno Schmid, Belp, Switzerland (cases 5, 9, and 10); Dr Markus Salm, Bern, Switzerland (case 6); Dr Adrian Zbinden, Solothurn, Switzerland (case 7); Dr Chris Hart, Bern, Switzerland (cases 8 and 12); Dr Konrad Rüeger, Lenzburg, Switzerland (case 11); Dr Roland Spahr, Bern, Switzerland (case 13); Dr Domagoj Stojan, Biel, Switzerland (case 14).

Case 1 Standard implant placement, distal extension situation in the mandible.

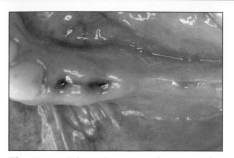

Fig 7-1a Edentulous quadrant in the left side of the mandible. The two premolars were removed 8 weeks earlier. Placement of three implants is planned for the first premolar and first and second molar sites.

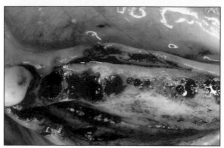

Fig 7-1b The crest is smoothed, and the implant positions are marked in the first and second molar sites with a small round bur.

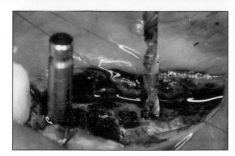

Fig 7-1c Standard implant site preparation with spiral drills of increasing diameter. The first 2.2-mm pilot drill is used here for the first molar implant site.

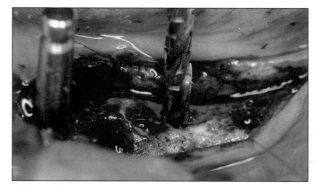

Fig 7-1d Implant site preparation continues with the second 2.8-mm spiral drill. A depth gauge in the premolar site is used to parallel both implant axes.

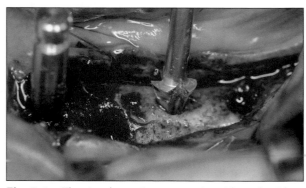

Fig 7-1e The implant site access is widened with a small-profile drill in preparation for the next spiral drill.

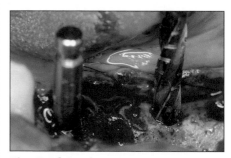

Fig 7-1f Implant site preparation is completed with a 3.5-mm spiral drill. Since the bone has rather low density, pretapping is not necessary.

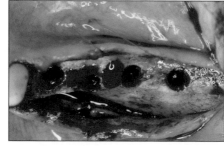

Fig 7-1g Occlusal view following implant site preparation.

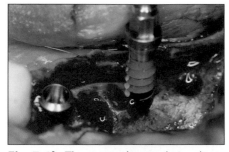

Fig 7-1h Three regular neck implants with a sand-blasted, large grit, acid-etched (SLA) surface are placed and achieve good primary stability.

▶

Fig 7-1i Following implant placement, healing caps are placed to extend the implants above the mucosal level.

Fig 7-1j The wound margins are precisely adapted and secured in place with several interrupted single sutures. Since this is a posterior site, nonsubmerged healing can be used.

Fig 7-1k One week following surgery, the soft tissue has healed enough for suture removal.

Fig 7-1l After 6 weeks, the soft tissue healing is complete, and the implants are sufficiently integrated for restoration with a fixed partial denture.

Fig 7-1m Definitive cemented fixed partial denture. The clinical status at the 8-year follow-up shows healthy peri-implant soft tissues.

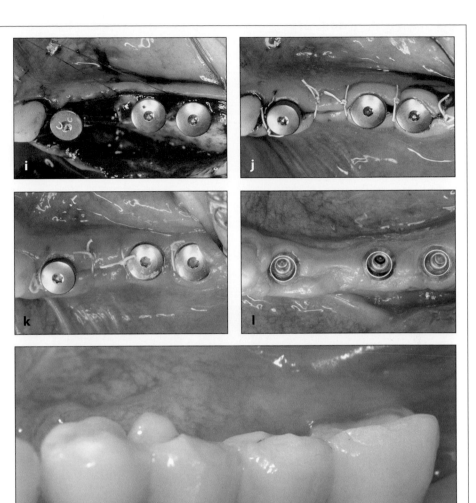

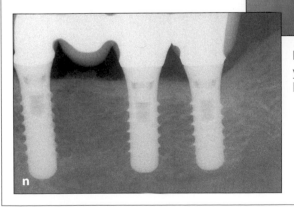

Fig 7-1n Periapical radiograph at the 8-year follow-up. The peri-implant alveolar bone crest levels are stable.

Case 2   Standard implant placement, single tooth gap in the posterior mandible.

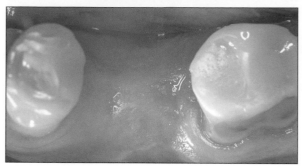

Fig 7-2a Missing first molar in the left side of the mandible. The gap size and crest width are sufficient to accommodate a wide neck implant.

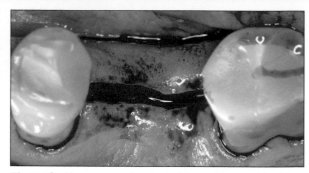

Fig 7-2b The surgery begins with a midcrestal incision without releasing incisions. The limited flap elevation will result in only minor postoperative pain and swelling.

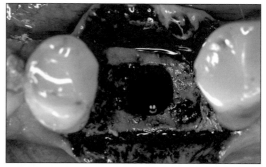

Fig 7-2c The buccal and lingual bony walls are intact after preparation of the implant site.

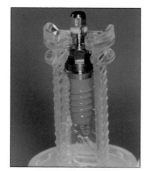

Fig 7-2d To preserve its hydrophylic, "SLActive" surface, the wide neck implant is kept in an electrolyte solution.

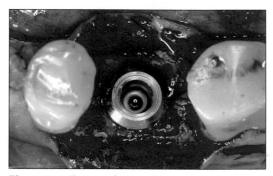

Fig 7-2e The implant achieves excellent primary stability, which is documented by an implant stability quotient (ISQ) of 80.

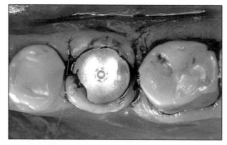

Fig 7-2f The wound margins are adapted around the 3-mm healing cap. The soft tissues are secured with two interrupted sutures of 5-0 suture material, allowing for nonsubmerged healing.

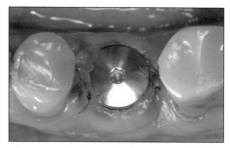

Fig 7-2g One week following surgery, soft tissue healing has progressed sufficiently for suture removal.

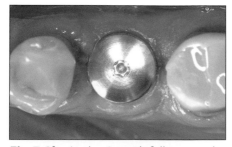

Fig 7-2h At the 3-week follow-up, the peri-implant soft tissues are healed and the healing cap can be removed.

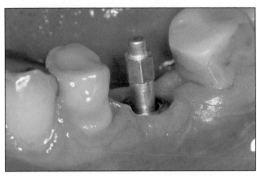

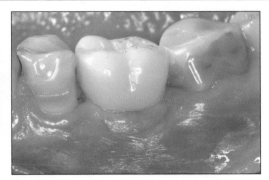

Fig 7-2i Implant stability is measured with resonance frequency analysis (RFA).

Fig 7-2j An ISQ of 83 indicates sufficient anchorage for early implant loading. As part of a prospective clinical study, the implant is loaded at day 21 with a provisional acrylic crown. The crown is in full occlusal contact.

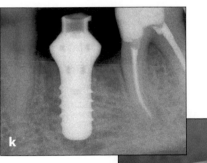

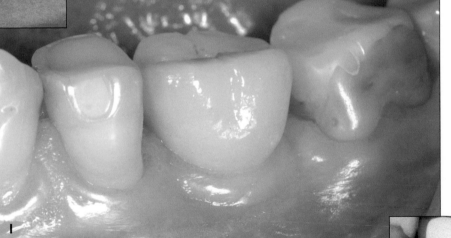

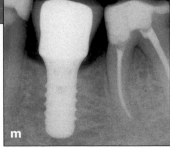

Fig 7-2k Periapical radiograph showing the well-integrated wide neck implant and the titanium coping base of the provisional crown.

Fig 7-2l Definitive cemented crown with healthy peri-implant soft tissue at the 1-year follow-up.

Fig 7-2m Periapical radiograph showing a well-integrated implant with stable alveolar bone crest levels at the 1-year follow-up.

Case 3 Standard implant placement, extended edentulous gap in the posterior mandible.

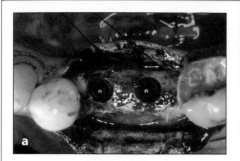

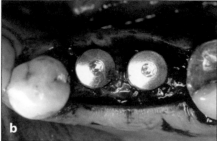

Fig 7-3a Two missing teeth in the left side of the mandible. Both sites are prepared for placement of regular neck implants.

Fig 7-3b After the implants are placed, the wound margins are approximated to the implant shoulders to determine the best technique for soft tissue closure.

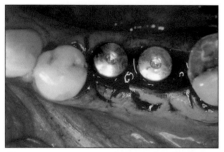

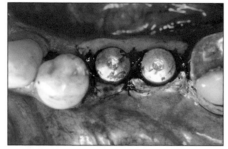

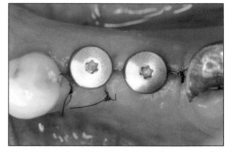

Fig 7-3c Two small pedicle flaps are prepared into the buccal wound margin. One is rotated into the interimplant space and the other between the distal implant and the adjacent tooth.

Fig 7-3d Following rotation of the pedicle flaps, the tension-free wound margins are adapted and secured with three interrupted sutures of 5-0 suture material.

Fig 7-3e At the 1-week follow-up, the soft tissue healing is sufficient to allow suture removal.

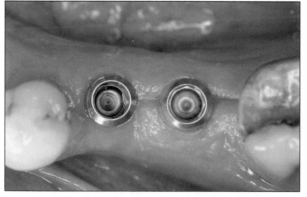

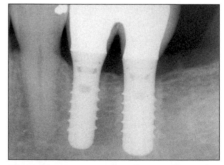

Fig 7-3f After 6 weeks of healing, the peri-implant soft tissues are well healed and healthy. The implants are ready for restoration.

Fig 7-3g Periapical radiograph at the 3-year follow-up. The alveolar bone levels around both implants are stable. The adjacent molar has been extracted since the last examination.

Case 4 Standard implant placement and soft tissue grafting in the posterior mandible.

Fig 7-4a Two implants are placed in the left side of the mandible and demonstrate good primary stability. Healing caps are placed to extend the implants above the soft tissue level.

Fig 7-4b Full thickness soft tissue graft harvested from the retromolar area and trimmed to the desired dimensions with a 5-mm tissue punch.

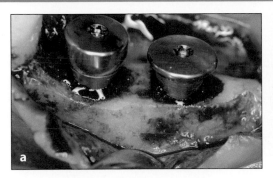
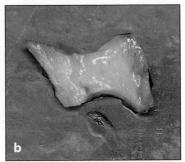

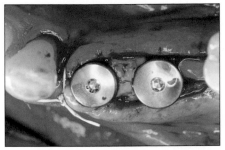
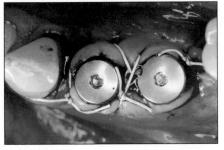
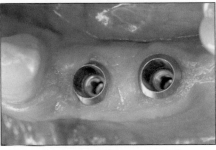

Fig 7-4c The graft is placed in the inter-implant space. Suturing begins at the mesial papilla to stabilize the wound margins.

Fig 7-4d Suturing continues with a crossed mattress suture to secure the wound margins and the soft tissue graft.

Fig 7-4e Clinical situation following healing. The peri-implant soft tissues appear healthy and show a wide band of buccal keratinized mucosa.

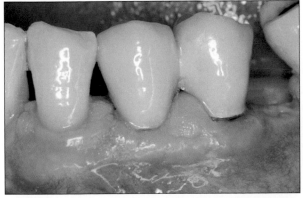
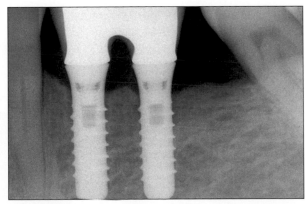

Fig 7-4f Follow-up view of the definitive restoration 5 years after implant placement. The restorative dentist splinted the two single crowns, which would not be done today.

Fig 7-4g Periapical radiograph at the 5-year follow-up. The crestal bone levels are stable. Splinting of the crowns led to an inaccurate fit between the implant shoulders and crown margins.

Case 5 Standard implant placement, distal extension situation in the maxilla.

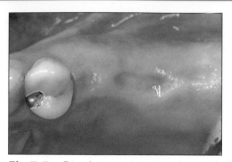

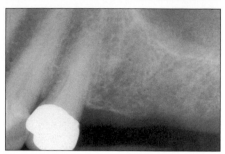

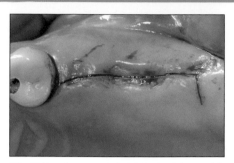

Fig 7-5a Distal extension situation with a missing second premolar and first molar in the maxilla. Crest width is sufficient for implant placement.

Fig 7-5b Preoperative radiograph showing sufficient alveolar bone height for the placement of a 10-mm implant in the premolar site and a 6-mm implant in the molar site.

Fig 7-5c Surgery is initiated with a midcrestal incision.

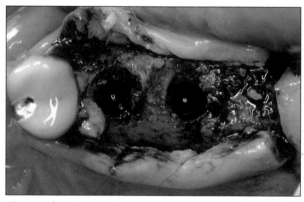

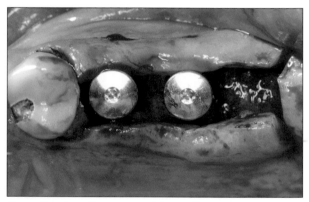

Fig 7-5d Following flap elevation and smoothing of the alveolar crest, both implant sites are prepared for appropriate prosthetic positioning. The wide alveolar crest allows for placement of two wide body implants.

Fig 7-5e Both implants achieve adequate primary stability. Following the placement of healing caps, the wound margins are adapted.

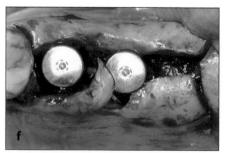

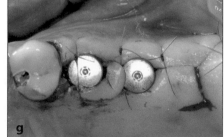

Fig 7-5f To avoid a gingivectomy on the buccal aspect, Palacci flaps are prepared into the palatal wound margin and rotated in proximally.

Fig 7-5g This technique allows precise, tension-free wound closure for nonsubmerged healing. The wound margins are secured with several interrupted single sutures of 5-0 suture material.

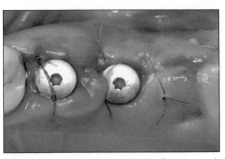

Fig 7-5h Clinical status at the 1-week follow-up, demonstrating sufficient soft tissue healing for suture removal.

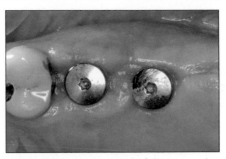

Fig 7-5i At the 4-week follow-up, the implants demonstrate favorable stability.

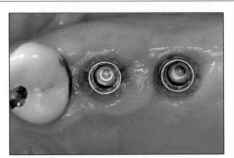

Fig 7-5j Eight weeks after surgery, the peri-implant soft tissues are nicely healed without evidence of inflammation. Both implants are well integrated and ready for restoration.

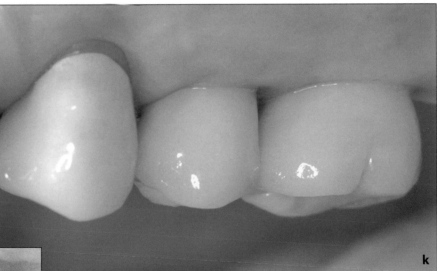

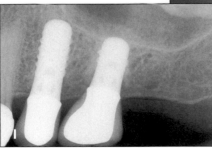

Fig 7-5k Clinical status at the 2-year follow-up. Both implants have been restored with cemented single crowns.

Fig 7-5l Two-year follow-up radiograph showing well-integrated wide body implants. The restorative dentist chose not to splint the crowns.

Case 6 **Standard implant placement, extended edentulous gap in the posterior maxilla.**

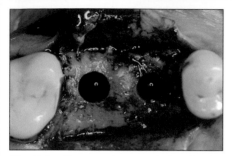

Fig 7-6a Two teeth are missing in the right posterior quadrant of the maxilla. Following a midcrestal incision and flap elevation, the implant site is prepared for appropriate prosthetic positioning.

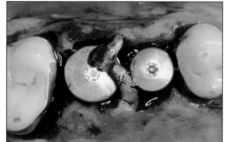

Fig 7-6b Following placement of two SLA-surfaced standard implants and 3-mm healing caps, the wound margins are adapted to the implant shoulders. In this case, small pedicle flaps are prepared to allow tension-free wound closure around the implants.

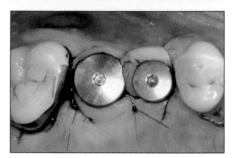

Fig 7-6c The wound margins are secured with three interrupted single sutures.

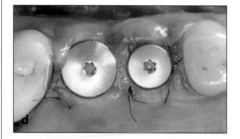

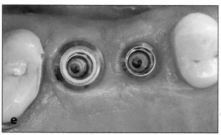

Fig 7-6d After 1 week, soft tissue healing has progressed and the sutures can be removed.

Fig 7-6e Six-week follow-up view showing excellent soft tissue healing. Both implants are well integrated and demonstrate favorable stability.

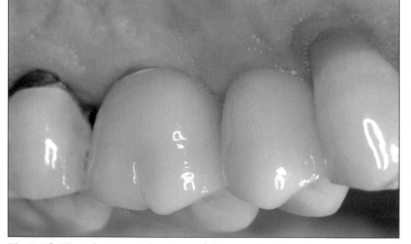

Fig 7-6f Clinical status at the 4-year follow-up. Both implants are restored with cemented ceramometal crowns without splinting.

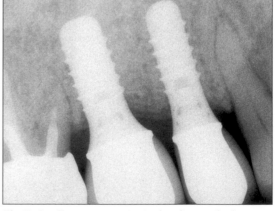

Fig 7-6g Four-year periapical radiograph showing well-integrated implants with stable alveolar bone levels.

Case 7 Standard implant placement with a periosteal pedicle flap in the posterior maxilla.

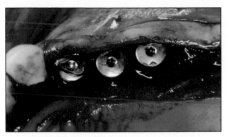

Fig 7-7a Distal extension situation in the left side of the maxilla. To obtain keratinized mucosa on the buccal aspect, a palatal incision was made, exposing the bone surface on the palatal aspect. Three titanium plasma-sprayed standard implants have been placed.

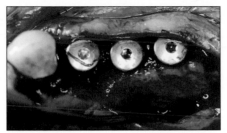

Fig 7-7b To cover the exposed bone surface, sharp dissection of the internal palatal mucosa is performed to prepare a pedicle-like periosteal flap, which obtains its blood supply from the mesial aspect. The periosteal flap is rotated toward the exposed palatal crest.

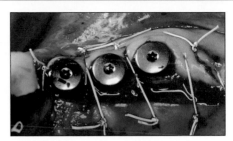

Fig 7-7c The periosteal flap and overlying mucosal flap are secured with several deep interrupted single sutures.

Fig 7-7d Two weeks after surgery, the periosteal flap is healing by secondary intention.

Fig 7-7e At the 3-month follow-up, the palatal mucosa is well healed and fully keratinized. The implants are ready to be restored.

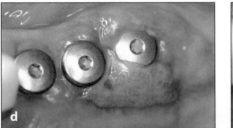
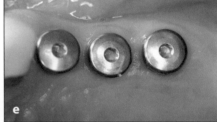

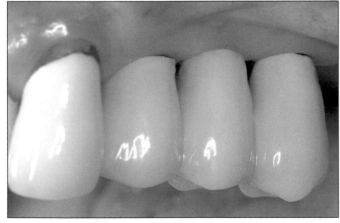

Fig 7-7f Clinical status at the 10-year follow-up. A 3-mm band of keratinized mucosa is evident on the buccal aspect, with no sign of inflammation. The three splinted crowns provide good masticatory function.

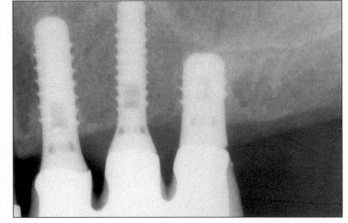

Fig 7-7g Periapical radiograph after 10 years of function showing excellent implant integration in the stable alveolar bone, including the 6-mm implant in the molar site.

Case 8 **Standard implant placement, single tooth gap in the posterior maxilla.**

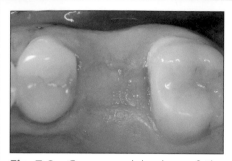

Fig 7-8a Gap caused by loss of the maxillary left first molar. Gap size, crest width, and alveolar bone height are sufficient to accommodate a 10-mm with a "SLActive" surface wide neck implant.

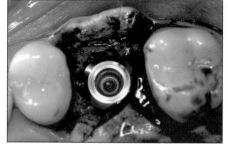

Fig 7-8b Implant placement achieves good primary stability with an ISQ of 70.

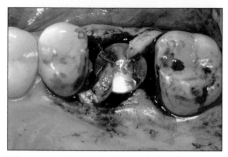

Fig 7-8c Two small pedicle flaps are prepared for a precise, tension-free adaptation of the wound margins.

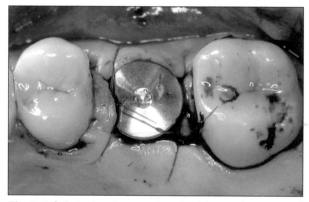

Fig 7-8d Suturing is completed with two interrupted single sutures of 5-0 suture material.

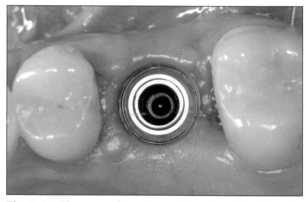

Fig 7-8e Three-week postoperative view showing the nicely healing soft tissue.

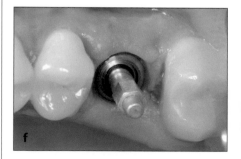

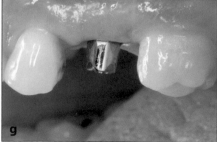

Fig 7-8f The implant demonstrates favorable stability. A magnetic post is placed to perform an RFA; the ISQ registers 72, indicating that the implant is ready for restoration.

Fig 7-8g One week later, a solid abutment is placed in preparation for a cemented single crown.

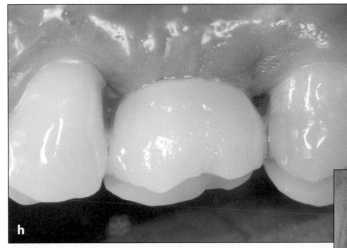

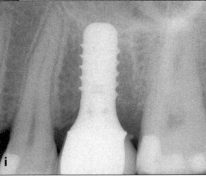

Fig 7-8h At day 28, the definitive restoration is cemented in place.

Fig 7-8i Periapical radiograph showing a well-integrated 10-mm wide neck implant with a cemented crown.

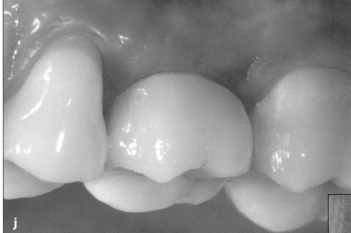

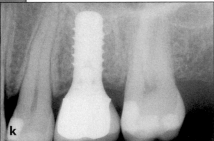

Fig 7-8j At the 4-month follow-up, healthy mucosa signals that the peri-implant soft tissues have adapted to the implant-borne crown.

Fig 7-8k Four-month follow-up periapical radiograph showing a well-integrated implant with normal peri-implant alveolar bone levels.

Case 9 **Standard implant placement with connective tissue grafting, single tooth gap in the anterior maxilla.**

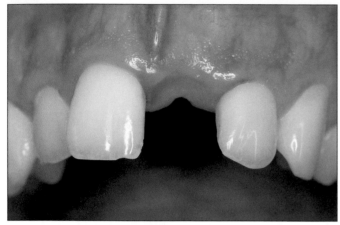

Fig 7-9a Missing central incisor in the anterior maxilla. Gap size, crest width, and alveolar bone height are sufficient to accommodate a 12-mm standard plus implant.

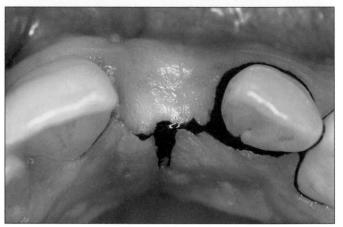

Fig 7-9b A crestal incision is made from a palatal approach to avoid a scar line in the area of future papillae.

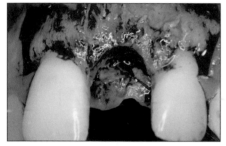

Fig 7-9c Releasing incisions are made at distal line angles, and the mucoperiosteal flap is elevated. The alveolar crest is carefully smoothed into a scallop shape without touching the bone in proximal areas.

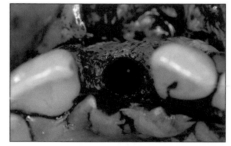

Fig 7-9d The bony wall on the facial aspect remains intact following implant site preparation.

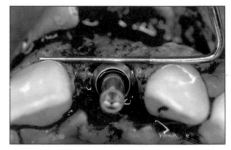

Fig 7-9e The implant is placed slightly palatal in a correct orofacial position as indicated by the periodontal probe.

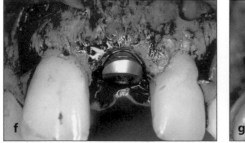

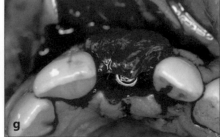

Fig 7-9f The implant is well positioned coronoapically and mesiodistally. A healing cap with a beveled design is placed on the implant.

Fig 7-9g To improve the esthetic contour of the facial soft tissues, a connective tissue graft is harvested from the palate and positioned on the facial aspect of the implant site.

Fig 7-9h The graft is secured to the mucoperiosteal flap with a mattress suture.

Fig 7-9i The periosteum is released, and interrupted single sutures allow for a tension-free flap closure and submerged healing.

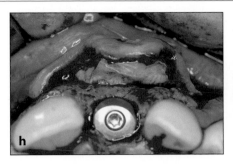

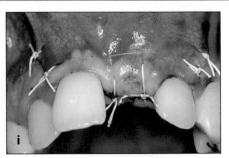

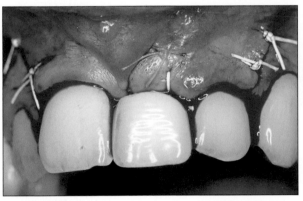

Fig 7-9j The existing removable partial denture is trimmed to prevent excessive pressure during soft tissue healing and repositioned over the surgical site.

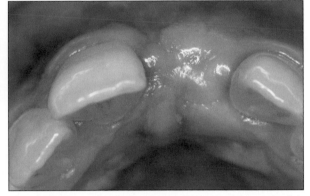

Fig 7-9k Completely healed soft tissues 6 weeks following implant placement.

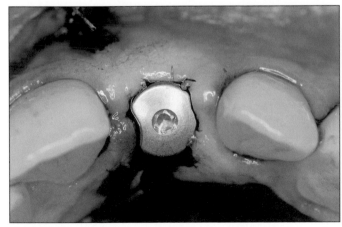

Fig 7-9l The implant is exposed with a punch technique using a 12b blade. The short healing cap is replaced by a longer healing cap to shape the transmucosal tunnel.

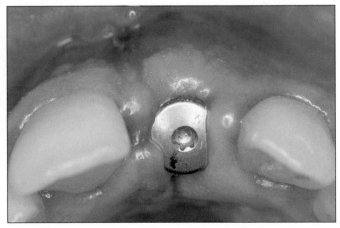

Fig 7-9m Soft tissue healing a few days after the uncovering surgery.

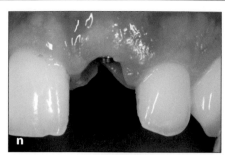

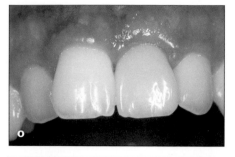

Fig 7-9n Facial view prior to provisional restoration.

Fig 7-9o Provisional acrylic crown with a titanium coping base.

Fig 7-9p Within a few months, the facial soft tissues have been nicely contoured by the shape of the provisional crown.

Fig 7-9q Definitive restoration with a screw-retained ceramometal crown. The 10-year follow-up demonstrates healthy and stable peri-implant soft tissues.

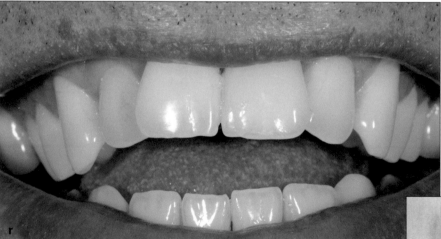

Fig 7-9r The pleasing esthetic treatment outcome is confirmed when the patient is smiling.

Fig 7-9s Periapical radiograph at the 10-year follow-up demonstrating stable peri-implant crestal bone levels.

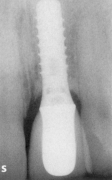

Case 10 Implant placement with simultaneous guided bone regeneration, apical fenestration defect.

Fig 7-10a Missing lateral incisor in the anterior maxilla. Gap size, crest width, and bone height are sufficient to accommodate a 12-mm narrow neck implant.

Fig 7-10b Elevation of a mucoperiosteal flap confirms the crest width and reveals an evident facial undercut.

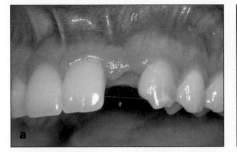
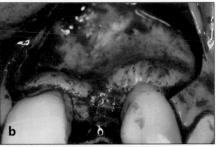

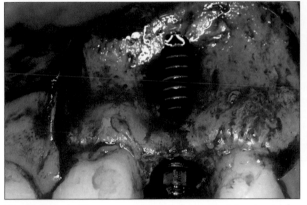
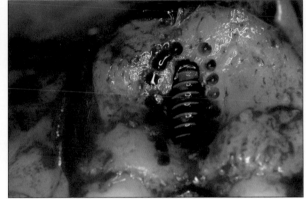

Fig 7-10c A 12-mm narrow neck implant is placed for appropriate prosthetic positioning. The apical fenestration defect requires simultaneous bone augmentation with a guided bone regeneration (GBR) procedure.

Fig 7-10d The peri-implant cortical bone is perforated with a small round bur to open the marrow cavity and stimulate the ingrowth of blood vessels into the coagulum.

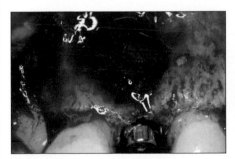
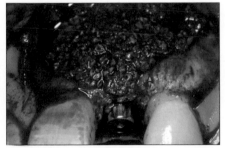
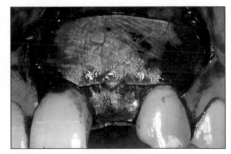

Fig 7-10e The exposed implant surface is covered with autogenous bone chips that have been soaked in blood. The bone chips were harvested at the nasal spine with a flat chisel.

Fig 7-10f The bone chips are covered with bone filler to improve the volume of the facial bone. Deproteinized bovine bone mineral (DBBM) has excellent biocompatibility and a low substitution rate.

Fig 7-10g The graft is covered with a resorbable collagen membrane, which serves as temporary barrier to keep the augmentation material in place. A double-layer technique improves the membrane stability.

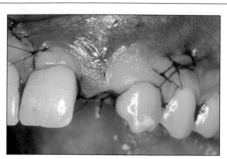

Fig 7-10h The periosteum is released, and a tension-free primary wound closure allows for submerged healing.

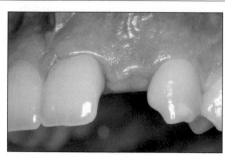

Fig 7-10i Clinical status after 2 months.

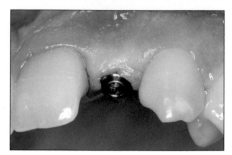

Fig 7-10j Uncovering surgery is accomplished from a palatal approach using a punch technique. The small healing cap is replaced with a longer 3.5-mm healing cap.

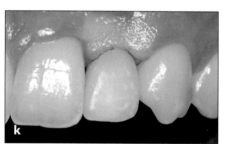

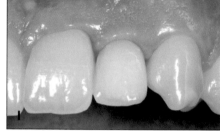

Fig 7-10k Provisional acrylic crown with a titanium coping base. The peri-implant soft tissues will need to adapt to the crown contour, as indicated by the soft tissue blanching.

Fig 7-10l Definitive restoration with a screw-retained ceramometal crown. The clinical status at 18 months demonstrates healthy and well-positioned soft tissues.

Fig 7-10m The esthetic result is pleasing when the patient smiles.

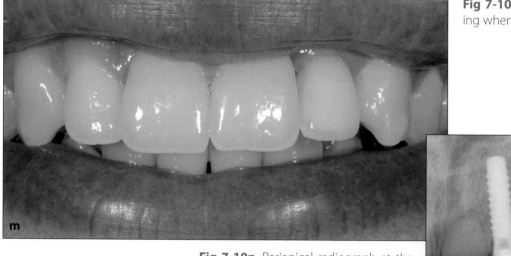

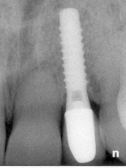

Fig 7-10n Periapical radiograph at the 18-month follow-up, demonstrating stable peri-implant bone levels.

Case 11 Implant placement with simultaneous guided bone regeneration, crestal dehiscence defect.

Fig 7-11a Single-tooth gap with a missing central incisor. Eight weeks earlier a low-trauma extraction without flap elevation was performed by the referring dentist. The 62-year-old female patient has been successfully treated for periodontal disease.

Fig 7-11b Elevation of a mucoperiosteal flap reveals a craterlike bone defect in the extraction site and vertical bone loss at adjacent teeth due to periodontal disease.

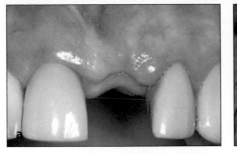

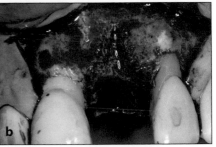

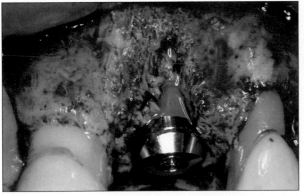

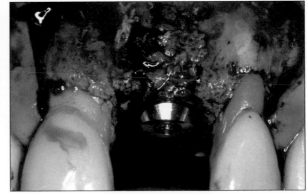

Fig 7-11c A 12-mm standard plus implant and a beveled healing cap are placed for appropriate prosthetic positioning. The crestal dehiscence defect has a favorable two-wall configuration and requires simultaneous bone augmentation with GBR.

Fig 7-11d Locally harvested autogenous bone chips fill the crestal bone defect and cover the exposed titanium implant surface. The autografts will encourage new bone formation in the area of the defect.

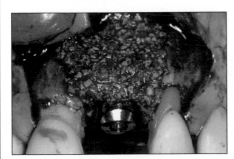

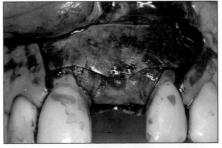

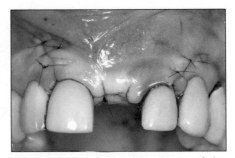

Fig 7-11e DBBM granules build up the facial bone volume. A convex contour is achieved for the alveolar process using this low-substitution bone filler.

Fig 7-11f The bone filler is covered with a resorbable collagen membrane, which serves as temporary barrier.

Fig 7-11g Following the release of the periosteum, a tension-free primary wound closure allows for submerged healing. The local bone anatomy is clearly more convex.

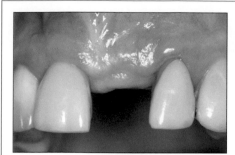

Fig 7-11h After 10 weeks, the surgical site is ready for uncovering surgery.

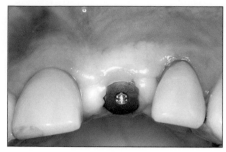

Fig 7-11i Uncovering surgery is accomplished from a palatal approach with a punch technique. A longer healing cap creates some pressure on facial soft tissues, as indicated by the mucosal blanching.

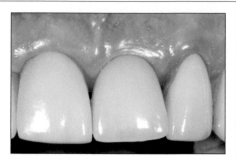

Fig 7-11j Clinical status with a provisional acrylic crown at the 2-year examination. The provisional restoration has remained in place longer than anticipated.

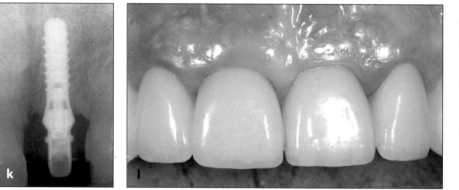

Fig 7-11k Periapical radiograph at the 2-year follow-up showing the titanium coping of the provisional crown.

Fig 7-11l Definitive screw-retained ceramometal crown at the 4-year follow-up. The adjacent teeth have been restored with all-ceramic crowns by the referring dentist.

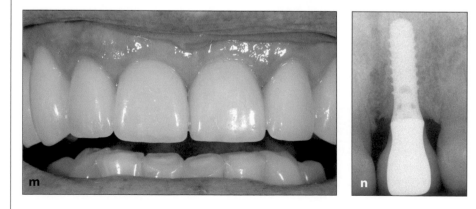

Fig 7-11m The high lip line of the patient's smile shows off the excellent esthetics at the 4-year examination. A harmonious gingival scallop with symmetric papillae contributes significantly to the esthetic result.

Fig 7-11n Periapical radiograph at the 4-year follow-up demonstrating stable peri-implant crestal bone levels.

Case 12 Implant placement with simultaneous guided bone regeneration, postextraction defect.

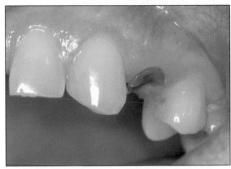

Fig 7-12a Remaining root of a first premolar in the left side of the maxilla. The root cannot be restored and requires extraction.

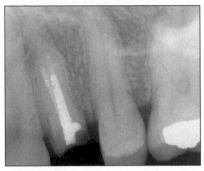

Fig 7-12b Periapical radiograph showing the remaining root. The bone height is sufficient for implant placement.

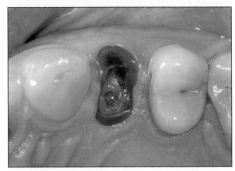

Fig 7-12c Occlusal view demonstrating adequate crest width.

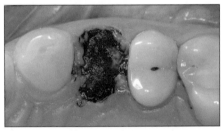

Fig 7-12d The root is carefully removed without flap elevation. Following debridement, the socket is filled with a collagen plug to stabilize the coagulum.

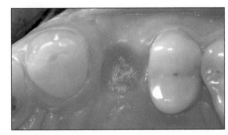

Fig 7-12e Four weeks after extraction, the soft tissues are well healed, and the site is ready for early implant placement.

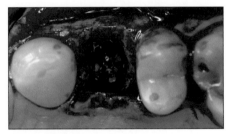

Fig 7-12f Flap elevation reveals an extraction socket defect and confirms the well-maintained crest width.

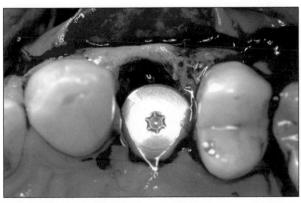

Fig 7-12g A tapered effect implant is placed slightly palatal within the extraction socket to optimize implant stability.

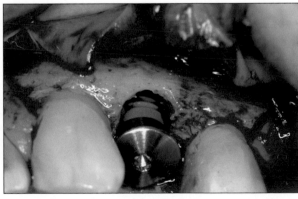

Fig 7-12h Facial view showing the minor crestal bone defect with a favorable two-wall morphology, which allows a simultaneous GBR procedure. The exposed implant surface is within the extraction socket.

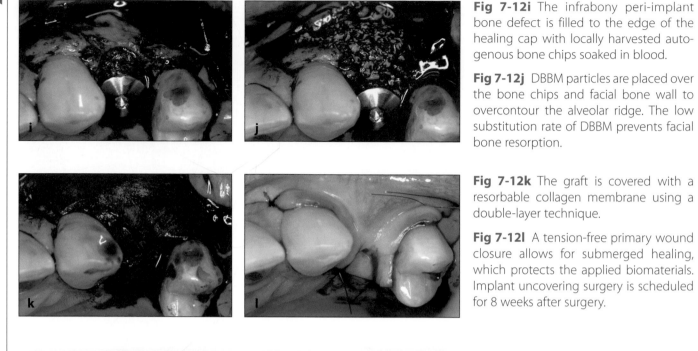

Fig 7-12i The infrabony peri-implant bone defect is filled to the edge of the healing cap with locally harvested autogenous bone chips soaked in blood.

Fig 7-12j DBBM particles are placed over the bone chips and facial bone wall to overcontour the alveolar ridge. The low substitution rate of DBBM prevents facial bone resorption.

Fig 7-12k The graft is covered with a resorbable collagen membrane using a double-layer technique.

Fig 7-12l A tension-free primary wound closure allows for submerged healing, which protects the applied biomaterials. Implant uncovering surgery is scheduled for 8 weeks after surgery.

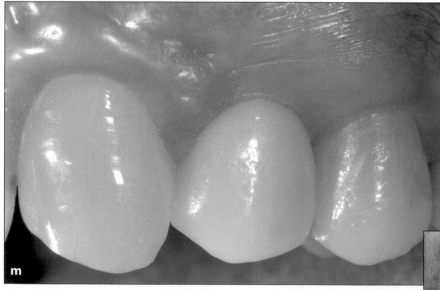

Fig 7-12m Clinical status 8 months after implant placement. The definitive ceramometal crown provides a pleasing esthetic result.

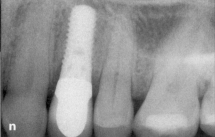

Fig 7-12n Periapical radiograph 8 months after implant placement. The implant is well integrated, although the alveolar bone has not yet fully remodeled at the crest level.

Case 13 Implant placement with simultaneous sinus floor elevation via lateral window technique.

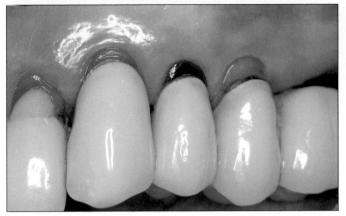

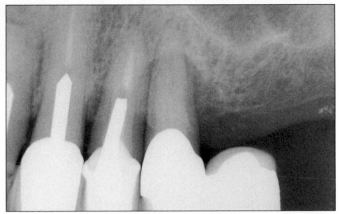

Fig 7-13a Clinical status of the left maxilla in an 85-year-old female patient. The patient wants a fixed restoration.

Fig 7-13b Periapical radiograph showing osteolytic lesions around both premolars and a bone height in the molar area between 5 and 6 mm. Extraction of both premolars is indicated.

Fig 7-13c The two premolars are carefully extracted without flap elevation. A period of two months is scheduled to allow for adequate soft tissue healing.

Fig 7-13d Two months after extraction, the soft tissues in the left maxilla are well healed.

Fig 7-13e Panoramic slice from a digital volume tomography scan showing the extraction sockets as well as the reduced bone height in the first molar site. To improve bone height in this area, and due to the oblique sinus floor anatomy, a sinus floor elevation is planned using the lateral window technique.

Fig 7-13f Clinical status following a midcrestal incision and elevation of a mucoperiosteal flap. Both premolar extraction sockets are visible, and the alveolar crest is fully intact in the first molar site.

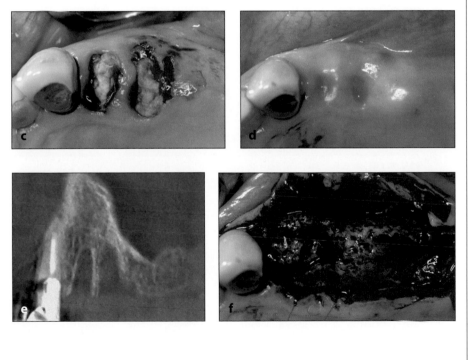

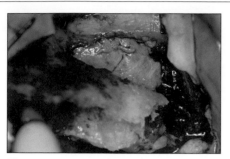

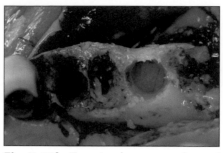

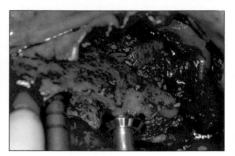

Fig 7-13g A window is prepared into the facial bone wall with diamond burs, and the sinus membrane is carefully mobilized from the inner surface of the sinus floor.

Fig 7-13h Two implants are planned for the first premolar and first molar sites. Visibility of the sinus membrane through the prepared molar site confirms the reduced bone height in the molar area.

Fig 7-13i A mixture of autogenous bone chips and DBBM particles is used to fill the space created by the sinus elevation. A 10-mm tapered effect implant is placed in the first molar site and achieves good primary stability due to its shape. The implant surface is partially exposed in the apical area.

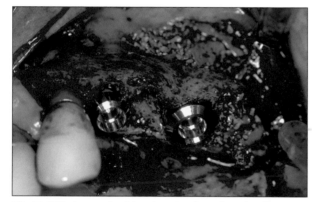

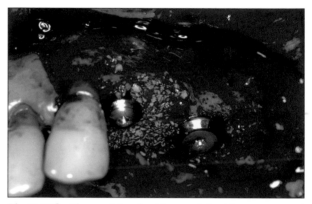

Fig 7-13j A standard implant is placed in the first premolar site, which exhibits a peri-implant bone defect. Additional DBBM particles are placed to cover the exposed implant surfaces.

Fig 7-13k The peri-implant bone defect is augmented with autografts and a superficial layer of DBBM particles.

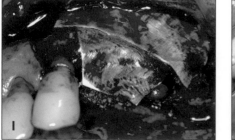

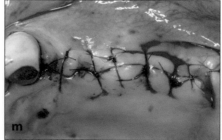

Fig 7-13l The graft is covered with a collagen membrane that has been soaked in blood. The double-layer technique improves the membrane stability.

Fig 7-13m Once the periosteum on the facial flap is released, a tension-free primary wound closure is achieved with several interrupted single sutures of 4-0 suture material.

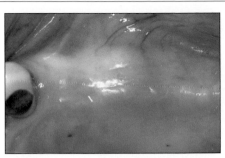

Fig 7-13n Four months after implant placement, the soft tissues are well healed.

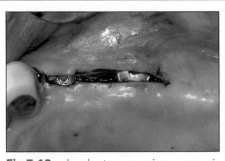

Fig 7-13o Implant uncovering surgery is accomplished with a slightly palatal crestal incision, which allows for some keratinized mucosa to be moved to the buccal aspect.

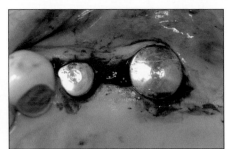

Fig 7-13p Short healing caps are replaced with longer 3-mm healing caps, and the keratinized mucosa is pushed to the buccal aspect.

Fig 7-13q Definitive restoration with a ceramometal, three-unit fixed partial denture. The clinical status 18 months following implant placement shows healthy peri-implant soft tissues and a pleasing esthetic outcome.

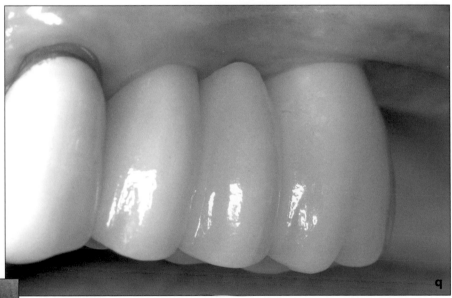

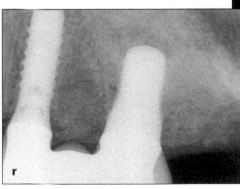

Fig 7-13r Eighteen-month periapical radiograph showing dense bone and stable bone crest levels.

Case 14 Implant placement with simultaneous sinus floor elevation via osteotome technique.

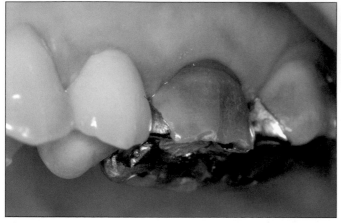

Fig 7-14a Discolored maxillary left first molar that is planned for extraction.

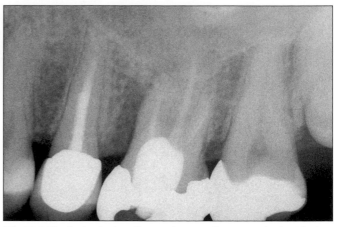

Fig 7-14b Periapical radiograph revealing a periapical lesion as well as reduced bone height, which is common in first molar sites.

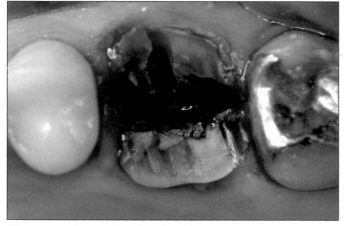

Fig 7-14c The tooth is carefully removed without flap elevation via separation of the three roots.

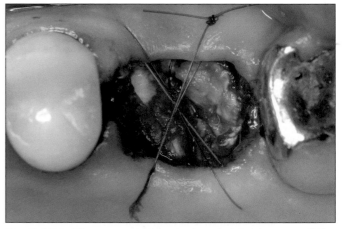

Fig 7-14d After a nose blow test and debridement of the socket, a collagen plug is secured in the socket with crossed mattress sutures to stabilize the coagulum.

Fig 7-14e Periapical radiograph after extraction showing the socket defect and a bone height of 7 mm. Four months of healing are planned.

Fig 7-14f After 4 months, the soft tissues are well healed, and there are no apparent signs of atrophy in the facial bone wall.

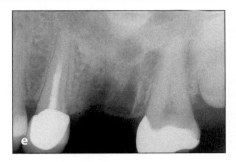

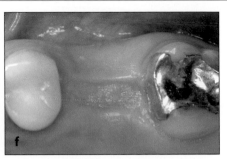

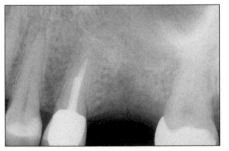

Fig 7-14g Periapical radiograph showing significant bone healing, which is essential for primary implant stability, given the reduced bone height.

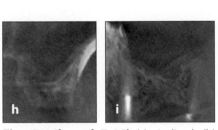

Figs 7-14h and 7-14i Mesiodistal *(h)* and orofacial *(i)* slices from a digital volume tomography scan. The rather flat anatomy of the sinus floor allows for use of the osteotome technique.

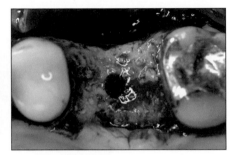

Fig 7-14j After a crestal incision is made and a facial flap elevated, the implant site is prepared with a 2.2-mm pilot drill to a depth of 5 mm.

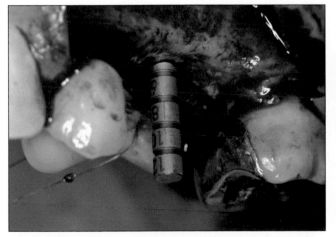

Fig 7-14k A 2.2-mm depth gauge placed in the implant site to verify depth.

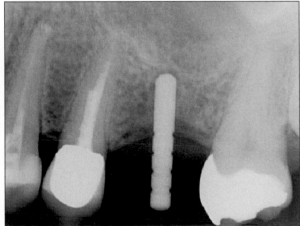

Fig 7-14l Intraoperative radiograph confirming the proximity of the tip of the depth gauge to the sinus floor. Implant positioning and axis are both correct.

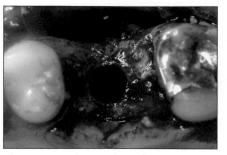

Fig 7-14m The implant site is prepared to a final diameter of 4.2 mm.

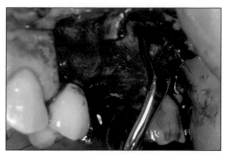

Fig 7-14n Autogenous bone chips are harvested from the facial bone wall with a bone scraper.

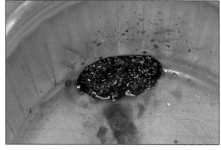

Fig 7-14o Autograft chips are mixed with DBBM particles in a ratio of 1:1 and soaked in blood.

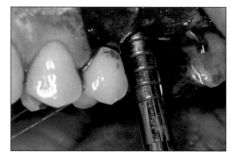

Fig 7-14p Following upfracture of the sinus floor, the composite graft is placed in the implant site, and the osteotome is used to push the graft apically. The nose blow test can confirm that the sinus membrane has not ruptured.

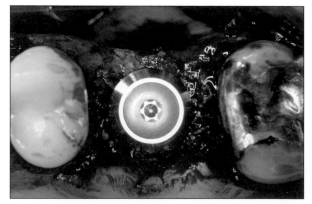

Fig 7-14q Composite graft is reapplied three to four times prior to placement of a 10-mm wide neck implant. The implant achieves good primary stability.

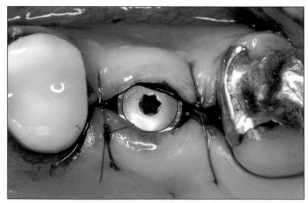

Fig 7-14r Following placement of a small healing cap, the wound margins are adapted and secured with two single interrupted sutures.

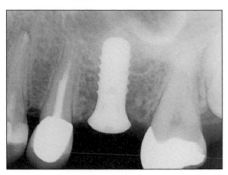

Fig 7-14s Postoperative radiograph showing good implant positioning as well as the 6-mm sinus floor elevation.

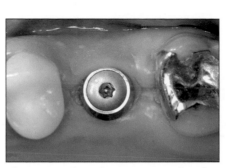

Fig 7-14t Clinical status 2 months after implant placement, demonstrating healthy peri-implant soft tissues.

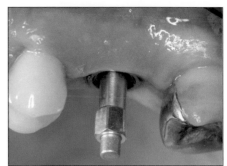

Fig 7-14u An ISQ of 75 confirms that the implant is well integrated and ready to be restored.

Fig 7-14v Clinical status at the 2-year follow-up. The cemented ceramometal crown is well integrated with the surrounding dentition, and the peri-implant soft tissues are healthy.

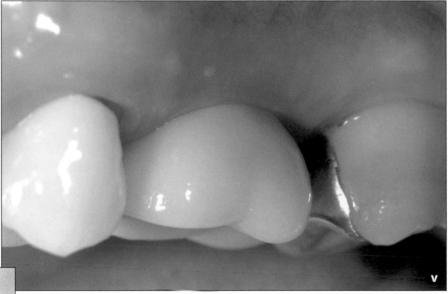

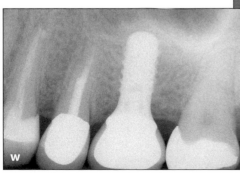

Fig 7-14w Periapical radiograph at the 2-year follow-up showing an integrated implant with well-remodeled periapical bone and stable crestal bone levels.

Suggested Reading

Buser D, Martin W, Belser UC. Optimizing esthetics for implant restorations in the anterior maxilla: Anatomic and surgical considerations. Int J Oral Maxillofac Implants 2004;19(suppl):43–61.

Buser D, Martin W, Belser UC. Surgical considerations with regard to single-tooth replacement in the esthetic zone. In: Buser D, Belser UC, Wismeijer D (eds). ITI Treatment Guide. Vol 1: Implant Therapy in the Esthetic Zone: Single-Tooth Replacements. Berlin: Quintessence, 2007: 26–37.

Buser D, von Arx T. Surgical procedures in partially edentulous patients with ITI implants. Clin Oral Implants Res 2000;11(1 suppl):83–100.

Jensen O (ed). The Sinus Bone Graft, ed 2. Chicago: Quintessence, 2006.

Palacci P, Ericsson I (eds). Esthetic Implant Dentistry: Soft and Hard Tissue Management. Chicago: Quintessence, 2001.

Sclar AG. Soft Tissue and Esthetic Considerations in Implant Therapy. Chicago: Quintessence, 2003.